STUDY GUIDE TO ACCOMPANY

Maternal and Neonatal Nursing Family-Centered Care
third edition

Katharyn A. May and Laura R. Mahlmeister

Cecilia M. Tiller, RN, DSN
Assistant Professor
Department of Parent-Child Nursing
Medical College of Georgia
Augusta, Georgia

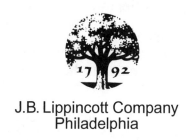

J.B. Lippincott Company
Philadelphia

Sponsoring Editor: Jennifer Brogan
Ancillary Coordinator: Doris Wray
Production Manager: Janet Greenwood
Compositor: Richard Hartley
Printer: Capital City Press

Copyright © 1994, by J. B. Lippincott Company. All rights reserved. No part of this book may be used or reproduced in any manner whatsoever without prior written permission except for brief quotations embodied in critical articles and reviews. Printed in the United States of America. For information write J. B. Lippincott Company, 227 East Washington Square, Philadelphia, Pennsylvania 19106.

ISBN 0-397-55124-X

6 4 2 1 3 5

Any procedure or practice described in this book should be applied by the healthcare practitioner under appropriate supervision in accordance with professional standards of care used with regard to the unique circumstances that apply in each practice situation. Care has been taken to confirm the accuracy of information presented and to describe generally accepted practices. However, the authors, editors, and publisher cannot accept any responsibility for errors or omissions or for any consequences from application of the information in this book and make no warranty express or implied with respect to the contents of the book.

Every effort has been made to ensure drug selections and dosages are in accordance with current recommendations and practice. Because of ongoing research, changes in government regulations, and the constant flow of information on drug therapy, reactions, and interactions, the reader is cautioned to check the package insert for each drug for interactions, dosages, warnings and precautions, particularly if the drug is new or infrequently used.

Preface

Health Care is changing dramatically. New knowledge and technology develop so quickly they push the boundaries of professional practice forward at an astonishing pace. In no other specialty is this change as obvious as in maternal-neonatal care. The professional nurse of today and tomorrow faces an almost overwhelming array of technological applications to care and is called on to assume increasing responsibilities. At the same time, the human aspect is still of the utmost importance in such an overwhelming life event.

This student **Study Guide to Accompany Maternal and Neonatal Nursing: Family-Centered Care**, Third Edition, provides exercises to assist you with learning and applying the critical information, concepts and principals presented in the text. The **Study Guide** is divided into chapters that correspond to those in the text. For the most part, each chapter in the Study Guide contains the following elements.

Chapter Summary:	A summary of the content in the textbook chapter.
Learning Objectives:	A list of learning goals that you will he able to meet after you read the textbook and work through the exercises in the Study Guide.
Application of Key Terms:	Matching exercises that ask you to identify the definitions of key terms.
Short Answer Exercise:	Questions that require you to supply missing information, list critical material, and demonstrate your knowledge of key chapter content.
Multiple Choice Exercise:	Questions that are designed specifically to allow you to identify and apply essential concepts to patient situations or in a clinical context.
True and False Exercises:	Questions that are answered by knowing whether the statement is true or false. If the answer is false, you are required to correct it so that it becomes true.
Matching Exercises:	Questions that address the meaning of key concepts.
Critical Thinking Exercises:	Questions and activities that require you to apply your new knowledge to real life nursing situations.

The various types of questions and exercises in the **Study Guide** are designed to help you better understand and apply the material presented in **Maternal and Neonatal Nursing: Family Centered Care,** Third Edition. Together, the text and the Study Guide will provide you with a useful foundation from which to build professional nursing practice.

Table of Contents

Preface		i
Chapter 1	Contemporary Maternal and Neonatal Care	1
Chapter 2	Conceptual Foundations of Maternal and Neonatal Nursing	5
Chapter 3	Challenges in Maternal and Neonatal Nursing	8
Chapter 4	Normal Reproductive Anatomy and Physiology	12
Chapter 5	Human Sexuality	19
Chapter 6	Women's Health Across the Life Span	24
Chapter 7	Fertility Management	30
Chapter 8	Individual and Family Adaptation to Pregnancy	40
Chapter 9	Adolescent Childbearing and Parenting	47
Chapter 10	Childbearing and Parenting After Age 35	53
Chapter 11	Physiologic Adaptations in Pregnancy	57
Chapter 12	The Genetic Code and Fetal Development	62
Chapter 13	Nursing Assessment of the Pregnant Woman	69
Chapter 14	Assessment of Fetal Well-Being	76
Chapter 15	Nursing Care of the Expectant Family	82
Chapter 16	Complications of Pregnancy	89
Chapter 17	Nutrition During Pregnancy	97
Chapter 18	Comprehensive Education for Childbirth	103
Chapter 19	The Process of Labor And Birth	108
Chapter 20	Nursing Care in Normal Labor	117
Chapter 21	Nursing Care in Normal Birth	125
Chapter 22	Monitoring the At-Risk Fetus	134
Chapter 23	Modifying Labor Patterns and Mode of Delivery	140
Chapter 24	Managing Pain During the Intrapartum and Postpartum Periods	146
Chapter 25	Nursing Care of the At-Risk family in the Perinatal Period	151
Chapter 26	Intrapartum Complications	156
Chapter 27	Perinatal High-Risk Challenges	165
Chapter 28	Nursing Care of the Family in the Postpartum Period	173
Chapter 29	Postpartum Complications	179

Chapter 30	Assessment of the Neonate	186
Chapter 31	Nursing Care of the Low-Risk Neonate	194
Chapter 32	Assessment of the At-Risk Neonate	200
Chapter 33	Nursing Care of the High-Risk Neonate	206
Chapter 34	Congenital Anomalies in the Neonate	214
Chapter 35	Maternal and Infant Nutrition	220
Chapter 36	Individual and Family Adaptation in the Year After Childbirth	224
Answer Key		229

UNIT I: INTRODUCTION TO MATERNAL AND NEONATAL CARE

CHAPTER 1

Contemporary Maternal and Neonatal Care

Overview

This chapter introduces the student to family-centered nursing care and begins with a brief overview of the historical influences upon perinatal nursing. Awareness of historical, social, and economic trends allows nurses to anticipate how changes will affect professional practice. Standards for perinatal nursing and the various roles of the perinatal nurse is governed by ethical, legal, and research findings and concerns.

Learning Objectives

After studying the material in this chapter, the student will be able to:

- Outline historical trends affecting the development of perinatal care in the United States.
- Identify social and economic trends affecting the current organization of perinatal care.
- Define family-centered perinatal nursing.
- Discuss the major principles underlying the philosophy of family-centered perinatal care.
- Discuss the nurse's role in establishing and maintaining family-centered perinatal care for childbearing families.

Application of Key Terms

Match the definitions in column two with the key terms in column one.

_____ 1. Diagnosis-related group (DRG)
_____ 2. Family-centered perinatal care
_____ 3. Neonatologist
_____ 4. Nurse Midwife
_____ 5. Perinatal period
_____ 6. Perinatologist

A. A registered nurse who has completed a specialized course of training.
B. Physician with special training in the care of the neonate
C. Period from the 28th week of gestation through the 28th day of life.
D. A strategy for controlling health care costs with predetermined reimbursement.
E. Delivery of quality health care that focuses on and accommodates both the physical and psychosocial needs of the family.
F. Obstetrician with special interest and experience with high-risk mothers and infants.

UNIT I: INTRODUCTION TO MATERNAL AND NEONATAL CARE

Short Answer Exercise of Critical Content

1. Describe five discoveries or inventions by physicians in the 16th and 17th centuries that set the stage for scientific progress.

    a.

    b.

    c.

    d.

    e.

2. List four out of six developments that contributed to the shift away from home birth to hospital care after 1900, and explain the influence of each.

    a.

    b.

    c.

    d.

3. List factors influencing delivery of perinatal care.

CONTEMPORARY MATERNAL AND NEONATAL CARE

Multiple Choice Exercise of Critical Content

Circle the most correct answer

1. The natural childbirth movement grew in strength and popularity in the late 1950s. The major strategy for these organizations was to:

    a. Take deliveries out of the hospital.

    b. Replace the nurse midwife in the delivery situation.

    c. Educate expectant parents.

    d. Make patient rights under the control of the physician.

2. As perinatal care has evolved and as technology has become more complex, the perinatal nurse has become a specialist. A good example of a nurse specialist would be:

    a. Staff nurse

    b. Nurse midwife

    c. Clinical nurse

    d. Office nurse

3. Many parents want to be together with their neonate in the first hours after birth. This practice is an example of what concept?

    a. Perinatal care

    b. Sibling preparation

    c. Family-centered care

    d. Nurse controlled care.

Matching Exercise of Critical Content

Match the following. Some answers may be used more than once. Some blanks have more than one answer.

_____ 1. 1935 Amendment to Title V of the Social Security Act.

_____ 2. The Sheppard-Towner Act of 1921.

_____ 3. Maternal and Infant Care (MIC) projects.

_____ 4. The Frontier Nursing Service

_____ 5. The Maternity Center Association in New York City.

A. Marked the first federal involvement in maternity care

B. Established in 1925 to provide care for families in Appalachia.

C. Provided funding for maternal-child health programs in response to priorities set by a national commission.

D. A charitable program founded in 1918 to care for poor women and children.

E. Emphasized comprehensive prenatal and infant care in public clinics.

F. Gave rise to nurse-midwifery in the United States.

UNIT I: INTRODUCTION TO MATERNAL AND NEONATAL CARE

True and False Exercise of Critical Content

The following statements require you to assess whether or not a practice is research-based. Indicate whether the statements are true or false. If the statement is false, rewrite it so that it is correct.

1. There is some fear of emotional distress and possible lawsuits by fathers who are in attendance at cesarean births; however, this is not supported in health care literature. (True/False).

2. Research has proven that sibling rivalry is lessened when the older child is present at the birth of the baby. (True/False).

3. Studies have documented the participation of siblings in the birth experience is emotionally stressful. (True/False).

4. Research shows that complication rates in home births are generally lower than complication rates in the hospital setting. (True/False).

Critical Thinking Exercises

1. Susan Jones, a 20 year old newly diagnosed pregnant married female, approaches you to discuss options for childbirth. Formulate a plan to explain childbirth options to Mrs. Jones.

2. Karen Smith is a new graduate of a baccalaureate program and has decided to continue her education in perinatal nursing. Explain the options she has and what type of education she should seek.

CHAPTER 2

Conceptual Foundations of Maternal and Neonatal Nursing

Overview

Characteristics of professional status address the knowledge base common to a professional group and the organizing frameworks within which these professionals practice. This chapter focuses on the use of an identifiable knowledge and theory base to plan and provide nursing care. Although many elements addressed in this chapter are common to all fields of nursing, some have particular importance in the care of childbearing families.

Learning Objectives

After studying the material in this chapter, the student will be able to:

- Discuss the advantages of using a conceptual framework in clinical practice
- Explain the concept of adaptation and discuss why adaptation theory may be useful in caring for childbearing families.
- Explain the nursing process and its relationship to the nursing care plan.
- List nursing diagnoses that may be applicable to the care of childbearing families.
- Describe managed care and explain how it is being used in the care of childbearing families.
- State the importance of teaching as a nursing strategy in perinatal care.

Application of Key Terms

Match the definitions in column two with the key terms in column one.

_____ 1. Theoretical or conceptual framework
_____ 2. Adaption
_____ 3. Nursing Diagnosis
_____ 4. Collaborative problems
_____ 5. Managed care
_____ 6. Case management
_____ 7. Managed care path
_____ 8. Expected Outcome

A. Controls the process of providing the care through the actions of a case manager.

B. A system that focuses on coordinating the activities of health professionals to address needs.

C. The capacity to modify behavior and to change the environment to meet needs.

D. A clinical judgment about an individual, family or community response to actual or potential problem.

E. Organizing tools available to a profession.

F. An expression of what is to be accomplished within a specified time period.

G. Show the expected progression of the patient from initiation of care through discharge.

H. Physiologic complications that have resulted or may result from pathophysiologic, treatment-related, and other situations.

Short Answer Exercise of Critical Content

1. Define the nursing process and relate the importance of its use for nursing practice with childbearing families.

2. Write a nursing diagnoses for the following problems.

    a. Constipation.

    b. New, first-time mother.

    c. Nausea and vomiting during first trimester.

    d. Birth of triplets.

3. List critical considerations the perinatal nurse must be aware of prior to teaching a client and her family.

CONCEPTUAL FOUNDATION OF MATERNAL AND NEONATAL NURSING

Multiple Choice Exercise of Critical Content

Circle the most correct answer.

1. The systematic collection, analysis, and reporting of new information is a definition of:

    a. Nursing Diagnosis
    b. Nursing Practice
    c. Nursing Education
    d. Nursing Research

2. Mrs. Kempter, 32 years old, has just delivered her fifth baby. You are admitting her to the postpartum floor and developing her plan of care. An appropriate nursing diagnosis would include which of the following?

    a. High risk for infection related to unprotected intercourse with multiple partners.
    b. Knowledge deficit related to lack of experience in caring for a newborn.
    c. Pain related to persistent afterbirth cramping because of number of pregnancies.
    d. High risk for altered parenting related to adolescent parenthood.

3. Mrs. Kempter requests pain medication for her discomfort. Thirty minutes after receiving the pain medication you find her asleep. You chart the results knowing this is what step of the nursing process?

    a. Assessment
    b. Nursing Diagnosis
    c. Planning and Implementation
    d. Evaluation

Critical Thinking Exercise

1. Sue, a 13 year old was just told she is pregnant. Generate a plan of care to assist her in adapting to the changes that will take place over the next eight months.

2. You find Mrs. Avery crying as you approach her bedside. You know she delivered her second baby boy yesterday. Apply the steps of the nursing process to discover her problem and to develop a plan of care.

CHAPTER 3

Challenges in Maternal and Neonatal Nursing

Overview

The challenges in perinatal care are considerable. The number of underserved people is increasing and health care needs of low-income and minority groups are growing. There is a move to reduce health care costs. Nurses must maintain a clear vision of the future and concentrate on goals to achieve optimal care for childbearing women and their families.

Learning Objectives

After studying the material in this chapter, the student should be able to:

- Discuss current rates of maternal and infant morbidity and mortality in the United States.

- Identify major factors contributing to maternal and infant morbidity and mortality.

- Describe some major challenges facing those engaged in perinatal care.

- List advanced practice roles in perinatal nursing and describe the activities associated with each nursing role.

- Identify factors that will have a dramatic effect on perinatal care and on perinatal nursing in the future.

CHALLENGES IN MATERNAL AND NEONATAL NURSING

Application of Key Terms

Match the definitions in column two with the key terms in column one.

_____ 1. Birth rate
_____ 2. Certified nurse midwife
_____ 3. Infant mortality rate
_____ 4. Maternal mortality rate
_____ 5. Morbidity rate
_____ 6. Neonatal mortality rate
_____ 7. Neonatal period
_____ 8. Nurse practitioner

A. A registered nurse with advanced clinical preparation.
B. Pertaining to the sickness rate.
C. Number of live births per year for each 1000 individuals in the population.
D. The time from birth through the first 28 days of life.
E. A registered nurse who has completed a specialized course of training.
F. Infant deaths per 1,000 live births prior to 28 days old.
G. Maternal deaths per 100,000 live births from complications of pregnancy, childbirth and postpartum.
H. Infant deaths from birth to 1 year of age per 1,000 live births.

Short Answer Exercise of Critical Content

1. Analyze the major maternal-infant health concerns in minority populations.

2. List at least three barriers to optimal maternity care.

   a.

   b.

   c.

3. Name the organization that establishes standards of practice of perinatal nursing.

UNIT I: CHALLENGES IN MATERNAL AND NEONATAL NURSING

4. Nurses function in a variety of roles in providing care to childbearing families. Define each of the following roles. Include educational background and scope of function.

   a. The Certified Nurse Midwife

   b. The Clinical Nurse Specialist

   c. The Nurse Practitioner in Women's Health

   d. Nurse Consultants

   e. The Nurse Scientist in Perinatal Nursing

Multiple Choice Exercise of Critical Content

Circle the most correct answer.

1. Progress with improvements in maternal-infant health indicators nationwide continues to be less than optimal. Some statistics indicate that:
   a. The racial gap is thought to have no influence upon infant survival.
   b. Infant death rates continue to be higher among African Americans than European Americans.
   c. Hispanic Americans make up 12% of the United States population and comprise the largest minority group.
   d. Asian and Pacific Islander Americans present no health threats to maternal infant well-being.

2. One factor that may limit the impact of perinatal nursing on the future health of the nation is the oversupply of physicians. What area has the largest supply of physicians?
   a. rural
   b. suburban
   c. metropolitan
   d. townships

3. Nurses working in labor and delivery are at risk for litigation. What is the most common cause?

   a. charting all events
   b. communicating information
   c. interpretation of fetal monitoring
   d. substandard care

True and False Exercise of Critical Care

The following statements require you to assess whether or not a practice is ethical. Indicate whether the statements are true or false. If the statement is false rewrite it so that it is correct.

1. If a pregnant woman refuses to have a cesarean section to produce a potentially viable fetus, there is nothing the health care provider can do. (True/False)

2. The contemporary problems of maternal substance abuse and maternal HIV infection make ethical challenges very pressing. (True/False)

3. The risk and benefits of a procedure during pregnancy, need only to concern the woman. (True/False)

Critical Thinking Exercises

1. Review newspapers and magazines for articles about recent advances or changes in the field of maternity care. Analyze these articles to determine if they focus on technological advances or "person-based" changes in care. Evaluate if these changes will benefit the majority of families or just a relatively small number of people.

2. A nurse has been summoned to court about a case in which a mother presented in labor and delivery complete and the nurse had to deliver the baby. Because of the rapid delivery the baby aspirated some amniotic fluid. The mother is suing the hospital and the physican for substandard care. Formulate a plan that the nurse can develop to present the facts in court. Decide what things were charted (or should have been charted) that would help the nurse defend the case provided for the woman.

UNIT II: DYNAMICS OF HUMAN REPRODUCTION

CHAPTER 4

Normal Reproductive Anatomy and Physiology

Overview

A sound understanding of male and female anatomy gives the nurse confidence in dealing with sensitive issues surrounding reproduction. The nurse's role in health promotion is an ideal way to dispel the myths and misinformation perpetuated by uninformed sources. This chapter addressed the normal anatomy and physiology of the male and female reproductive systems. Male and female hormones and their importance in maintaining a normal reproductive tract is also addressed.

Learning Objectives

After studying the material in this chapter, the student will be able to:

- Describe the differentiation process in fetal development.
- Demonstrate a basic understanding of the male and female reproductive tracts.
- Identify the structures making up the female internal and external genitalia, and describe their function.
- List the major female hormones and their function.
- Discuss the menstrual cycle, and identify phases of the cycle and the dominant hormones of each phase.

NORMAL REPRODUCTIVE ANATOMY AND PHYSIOLOGY

APPLICATION OF KEY TERMS

Match the definitions in column two with the key terms in column one

_____ 1. Copulation
_____ 2. Endometrium
_____ 3. Gonad
_____ 4. Gonadotropin
_____ 5. Invagination
_____ 6. Menarche
_____ 7. Menopause
_____ 8. Menstrual cycle
_____ 9. Menstruation
_____ 10. Oocyte
_____ 11. Ovary
_____ 12. Ovulation
_____ 13. Puberty
_____ 14. Spermatogenesis
_____ 15. Stroma

A. Formation of mature, functional spermatozoa.
B. First menstruation that marks the beginning of cyclic menstrual function.
C. Insertion of one part of a structure within a part of the same structure; to ensheathe.
D. Sexual intercourse.
E. Foundation or supporting tissues of an organ.
F. Hormones having a stimulating effect on the gonads.
G. Early primitive ovum before it has completely developed.
H. Cessation of menstruation; it is considered complete when menses has not occurred for a year.
I. Mucous membrane lining the uterus (during pregnancy it is known as the decidua).
J. Periodic ripening and rupture of the mature ovum from the ovarian follicle.
K. Physiologic cyclic bleeding that, in the absence of pregnancy, normally occurs monthly in women of reproductive age.
L. Male and female sex organs (testes and ovaries).
M. A hallmark of reproductive function in females associated with endocrine changes and cyclic menstruation.
N. Point at which a person is first capable of reproduction.
O. An almond-shaped organ that develops and produces ova and secretes sex hormones.

Short Answer Exercise of Critical Content

1. Although genetically sex is determined at conception, for the first 6 weeks of gestation the conceptus remains sexually undifferentiated. The external genitals of the male and female embryo begin to differentiate between the _____ week of development. The ovaries develop at approximately _____ weeks. The hormone _____ stimulates the development of the penis, scrotum, and prostate gland.

2. The testes direct the function of the male reproductive system. List the chief functions of the testes.

3. The male organ of copulation is the _____.

UNIT II: DYNAMICS OF HUMAN REPRODUCTION

4. The penis consist of two lateral, cavernous bodies called _____ and _____ and a central core of erectile tissue called _____ that encloses the urethra.

5. The enlarged conic structure at the distal end of the penis is called the _____.

6. Describe the function of the epididymis.

7. List and briefly describe the purpose of the male accessory gland.

8. The female's urinary meatus is located between the _____ and _____.

9. The female urethra is approximately _____ long and on either side of the urethral meatus are two small duct openings to the _____ glands.

10. The external area extending from the lower vaginal orifice to the rectum is called the _____.

11. List three functions of the vagina.

    a.

    b.

    c.

12. The mucosa of the vaginal wall, stimulated by estrogen, maintains the normal acidic environment between a pH of _____ to _____.

13. Identify the location and function of each of the following uterine ligaments:

Ligament	Location	Function
Broad Ligament		
Round Ligament		
Uterosacral Ligament		

14. List the functions of the graafian follicle.

    a.

    b.

    c.

    d.

15. The primary hormones of the female reproductive system include _____, _____, and the gonadotropin _____ and _____. What are the three important and interrelated functions of these hormones?

    a.

    b.

    c.

Multiples Choice Exercise of Critical Content

Circle the most correct answer:

A group of women are waiting in the clinic for their first prenatal visit. You are conducting a class about the anatomy and physiology of their own bodies.

1. One of the younger girls asks about infections. You explain that the body protects the female from some infections by maintaining a(n):
   a. Alkaline pH and smegma secreted from the clitoris
   b. Acidic pH and bacteriostatic cervical mucosa
   c. Neutral pH of 7.5 and bactericidal secretions of labia minora
   d. pH of 4 to 5 and secretions of the Skene's ducts.

2. One of the women asks which hormone causes ovulation. You respond by telling the women that _____ is responsible for ovulation.
   a. Estrogen
   b. Follicle-stimulating hormone (FSH)
   c. Luteinizing hormone (LH)
   d. Progesterone

3. You go on to describe the menstrual cycle and inform the women that the hormones responsible for the menstrual cycle are:
   a. Estrogen and progesterone
   b. Gonadotrophins
   c. Gonadotrophins and estrogen
   d. Gonadotropin, estrogen, and progesterone

4. Further explanation of the menstrual cycle continues. The hormones(s) responsible for maturation of the graafian follicle is(are):
   a. Follicle-stimulating hormone
   b. Luteinizing hormone
   c. Follicle-stimulating hormone and estrogen
   d. Follicle-stimulating hormone and progesterone

5. A function of the ovaries would include:
   a. Producing the luteinizing hormone
   b. Inhibiting the production of the primordial follicle
   c. Producing estrogen and progesterone, causing changes during menstrual cycle
   d. Producing hormones that are oxytocic in nature

NORMAL REPRODUCTIVE ANATOMY AND PHYSIOLOGY

6. One girl asks what Ovulation is. You define Ovulation as:
    a. Maturation of the graafian follicle
    b. Rupture of the graafian follicle
    c. Seepage of blood through the vagina
    d. The follicular phase of the menstrual cycle

7. You explain that ovulation occurs
    a. At the time of menstruation
    b. Approximately 14 days after the onset of menstruation
    c. Approximately 14 days before the onset of menstruation
    d. In the middle of the menstrual cycle

8. Which of the following are functions of testosterone:
    a. Regulates the metabolic process of carbohydrate metabolism
    b. Stimulates the secretion of F.S.H. and I.C.S.H.
    c. Development and maintenance of the male secondary sex characteristics
    d. Stimulates secretion of the Cowper's glands

Matching Exercise of Critical Content

Match the following. Some answers maybe used more than once. Some blanks have more than one answer.

_____ 1. False pelvis
_____ 2. True pelvis
_____ 3. Ischial tuberosities and spines
_____ 4. Pelvic inlet
_____ 5. Pelvic outlet

A. Lies below the linea terminalis
B. Marks the pelvic brim or entrance into true pelvis
C. Lies superior to the linea terminalis
D. Represents the shortest diameter of the pelvis
E. The last part of the bony pelvis bordered by the coccyx and symphysis pubs
F. Varies in size and is not of obstetric importance
G. Inferior strait
H. Consist of the ilium, ischium, pubis, sacrum, and coccyx
I. About 10.5 cm
J. Bordered at the back by the sacral promontory and front by the top of the symphysis pubs
K. About 9.5 to 11.5 cm
L. Superior strait, about 11.5 cm

True and False Exercise of Critical Content

The following statements require you to assess whether or not it is true or false. If the statement is false, rewrite it so that it is correct.

1. The male external genitalia include the penis and the scrotum. (True/False).

2. Sensory impulses to the glans penis are highly organized. Sexual sensations pass through the intereostal space. (True/False).

3. The subcutaneous fascia of the scrotal wall is made up of involuntary muscle fibers called the corpus spongiosum. (True/False).

4. The prostate gland secretes and stores sperm. (True/False).

5. The male reproductive system consists of the testes, or male gonads, which produce sperm; ducts that store or transport sperm; accessory glands that produce secretions constituting the semen; supporting structures; and the penis. (True/False).

Critical Thinking Exercises

1. Plan a class on the process of menstruation. How would you explain the process to a group of adolescents? Arrange a group of adolescents to whom you can teach the class.

2. Elizabeth is the teenage daughter of one of your friends. She knows you are a nurse and asks you to explain the anatomy and physiology of the male and female reproductive systems to her. Analyze her learning needs and develop a plan to teach her the anatomy and physiology of the male and female reproductive systems.

CHAPTER 5

Human Sexuality

Overview

Beliefs about pleasure in sexual activity and sexual activity during pregnancy have ranged from complete prohibition to lack of any restriction. The rationale and guidelines for restrictions of sexual activity during pregnancy have been inconsistent. Frequently, health professionals do not inquire about a woman's sexual concerns or questions because they lack the education that prepares them to do so comfortably. This chapter explores basic information about human sexuality as a foundation for understanding how sexuality may be affected by childbearing and the changes of pregnancy that can inhibit or enhance sexual feelings.

Learning Objectives

After studying the material in this chapter, the student will be able to:

- Discuss the concept of sexual health.
- Discuss the changes that occur for both women and men during sexual responses.
- Explain the four phases of the sexual response cycle.
- Describe how pregnancy results in changes in sexual response in the areas of desire, arousal, and orgasm.
- Identify issues of sexual concern for pregnant couples on the relative risks of intercourse during menstruation, pregnancy, the postpartum period, and breastfeeding.
- Offer specific suggestions to use when approaching sexual problems during pregnancy and postpartum.

Application of Key Terms

Match the definitions in column two with the key terms in column one.

1. Cunnilingus
2. Dyspareunia
3. Gender identity
4. Fellatio
5. Homophobia
6. Lesbian
7. Masturbation
8. Orgasm
9. Sexual orientation

A. A female homosexual.
B. Painful intercourse.
C. Induction of sexual excitement to self through manipulation of the genitals or other body parts.
D. Oral sexual stimulation of the female genitals.
E. The fear or dislike of homosexuals.
F. The recognition of self as heterosexual, homosexual, or bisexual.
G. Oral stimulation of the penis
H. The recognition of self as either male or female.
I. Culmination of sexual excitement.

UNIT II: DYNAMICS OF HUMAN REPRODUCTION

Short Answer Exercise of Critical Content

1. Masters and Johnson described the response cycle they observed in terms of four phases. List these phases in order and briefly describe each phase.

    a.

    b.

    c.

    d.

2. Describe changes in female organs during sexual response.

    a. Labia majora:

    b. Labia minora:

    c. Clitoris:

    d. Pelvic muscles:

    e. Vagina:

    f. Cervix and uterus:

    g. Breast:

3. Describe changes in male organs during sexual response.

   Penis:

   Scrotum and testes:

   Prostate:

   Seminal vesicles:

   Cowper's glands:

   Pelvic muscles:

Multiple Choice Exercise of Critical Content

Circle the most correct answer

1. Variations in sexual interest and activity during pregnancy are difficult to predict. A typical pattern of interest in sexual activity among women during pregnancy might include:
   a. A steady continuous increase in sexual interest throughout pregnancy.
   b. A steady decline in sexual interest throughout pregnancy.
   c. No changes from the prepregnant state.
   d. All of the above.

2. Which trimester does the fear of miscarriage create anxiety that can cause couples to avoid sexual expression?
   a. First Trimester
   b. Second Trimester
   c. Third Trimester
   d. None of the above

3. During the second trimester it may be necessary for the couple to assume a different position for the sexual act. What position might the health care provider recommend.
   a. Sidelying facing one another
   b. Woman on top facing partner's face
   c. Missionary position, male on top
   d. All of the above except C

4. Mrs. Jones is in her 30th week of gestation and asked the nurse if she should be having strong contractions after orgasm. You might reply with which of the following statements?

    a. You had better tell you physician and stop having orgasms.

    b. It would be better if you would try different positions so that you do not experience orgasm.

    c. The uterus may have one long sustained contraction after orgasm, lasting for a minute or more.

    d. You should continue to have orgasms so that you will go into labor.

5. Once a woman has delivered, it is wise for her to not resume the sexual act prior to:

    a. The first week postpartum

    b. Four to 6 weeks postpartum

    c. About two weeks postpartum

    d. When ever the couple feels ready

6. Karen is planning to breastfeed her infant. The health care provider could assist her by telling her:

    a. Breastfeeding adversely affects the sexual response

    b. The breast can leak or spurt milk during arousal and orgasm.

    c. The woman should stop breastfeeding if she has orgasms while nursing.

    d. Breastfeeding causes permanent changes in the sexual desire.

True and False Exercise of Critical Content

Circle true if the statement is correct; circle false if the statement is incorrect and provide corrective information in the space provided.

1. Slang words for genitals are better for children to learn. (True/False)

2. Infants should be discouraged from exploring their genitals. (True/False)

3. The primary goal of health professionals caring for clients who may have sexual concerns needs to be the promotion of sexual health. (True/False)

4. A child of nine does not need to know that menstruation and masturbation are a normal part of growing up. (True/False)

5. The health professional needs to use concrete concepts and language when discussing pregnancy prevention with an adolescent. (True/False)

HUMAN SEXUALITY

6. The most important task of adolescence is identity formation. (True/False)

7. The historic Kinsey research reported the capacity for orgasm in boys as young as five months and girls as young as four months. (True/False)

8. The orgasmic platform is an engorgement of the outer third of the vagina. (True/False)

9. The refractory period is a recovery time during which further orgasm or ejaculation is physiologically impossible. (True/False)

10. Nursing an infant is considered an effective birth control method because the hormonal changes are predictable. (True/False)

Critical Thinking Exercise

1. You are the nurse caring for June Johnson, a 23 year old new mother. She is being discharged home with her first baby. You are planning for her discharge. She voices concern about ever getting her body back to normal. Plan the content of your discharge teaching.

2. Mable Smith, a 19 year old, has just been told she is pregnant. You have to obtain a sexual history from her. Evaluate your feelings about sex. Formulate your approach to Ms. Smith. Use the Assessment Tool at the end of chapter 5 to develop your approach.

CHAPTER 6

Women's Health Across the Life Span

Overview

The field of women's health has emerged as an area of specialty practice in nursing. It is an outgrowth of nursing's historical concern for the welfare of women and their families and extends beyond the limits of the childbearing cycle. This chapter provides an overview of the factors that significantly affect the health of women. Common health concerns faced by women during young, middle, and older adulthood are discussed.

Learning Objectives

After studying the material in this chapter, the student will be able to:

- Describe how the factors of sexism and poverty directly and indirectly affect the health and well-being of women.
- Identify the five major causes of death in women.
- Explain breast cancer screening techniques and state how other women should be screened.
- Describe cervical screening techniques and state how often women should be screened.
- Discuss the major mental health concerns affecting women.
- List the most common sexually transmitted diseases in the United States and discuss modes of prevention, detection, and treatment.
- Summarize the major physiologic changes women experience with aging.
- Define menopause and list its signs and symptoms and current treatments.
- Discuss the relationship between menopause and osteoporosis.

WOMEN'S HEALTH ACROSS THE LIFE SPAN

Application of Key Terms

Match the definitions in column two with the key terms in column one

_____ 1. Cervical intraepithelial neoplasia
_____ 2. Cervicitis
_____ 3. Fibrocystic breast disease
_____ 4. Heterosexism
_____ 5. Hormone replacement therapy
_____ 6. Mammography
_____ 7. Metrorrhagia
_____ 8. Osteoporosis
_____ 9. Perimenopausal period
_____ 10. Vasomotor disturbance

A. An x-ray study of breast tissue used in the diagnosis of breast disease.

B. Abnormal condition of cell growth in the cervix, formerly called dysplasia, which is the precursor to carcinoma.

C. Bleeding from the uterus at any time other than the menstrual period; maybe caused by lesions of the cervix.

D. A serious disorder, partly due to estrogen decline, that increases porosity of bone as women age.

E. A condition which there are palpable lumps in the breast, usually painful and fluctuate with the menstrual cycle.

F. Inflammation of the uterine cervix.

G. Orientation toward the opposite sex.

H. Period of years during which women experience gradual transition from reproductive to non-reproductive status.

I. A hot flash/flush ; a sensation of heat in the face and neck, followed by marked sweating over the upper body.

J. Estrogen replacement therapy for prevention of troublesome menopausal conditions.

Short Answer Exercise of Critical Content

1. List five major causes of death in women.

   a.

   b.

   c.

   d.

   e.

2. Briefly discuss breast cancer screening techniques and state how often women should be screened.

3. Briefly discuss cervical screening techniques and state how often women should be screened.

4. Contrast the differences between Anorexia and Bulimia. Which age group do these disorders affect the most?

5. For women who have a uterus and who are on hormone replacement therapy, the estrogen is opposed by giving _____ for all or part of the cycle to prevent the increased risk of developing _____.

6. List information you would give to sexually active females in regard to vaginal infections and sexually transmitted diseases?

WOMEN'S HEALTH ACROSS THE LIFE SPAN

7. Complete the following in regard to the most common sexually transmitted diseases in the United States.

Disease	Treatment	Diagnosis
Chlamydia		
Herpes		
Trichomoniasis		
Condyloma		
Gonorrhea		
Syphilis		
HIV/AIDS		

Multiple Choice Exercise of Critical Content

Circle the most correct answer.

1. Women's health is an emerging specialty in nursing. It emphasizes:
   a. Care of the indigent only.
   b. Factors that affect health and well-being of women throughout their lives.
   c. Factor that affect health and well-being of women during reproductive years.
   d. Care of women with dependent children.

2. Depression has been identified as a major health concern of women. Depression in women occurs at a rate twice as high as men and is most common between the ages of:
   a. 25 and 30 years.
   b. 30 and 45 years.
   c. 25 and 44 years.
   d. 30 and 50 years.

3. While reviewing Kerri's clinical chart, you learn that she has a history of dysmenorrhea. This means that Kerri has:

   a. Bleeding between menstrual cycles.
   b. Excessively heavy menstrual flow.
   c. Irregular menstrual cycles.
   d. Painful menstrual periods.

4. Which of the following findings during a breast self-examination should Mrs. Zobler report to her health care provider?

   a. Difference in size between the breast.
   b. Silver colored stretch lines.
   c. Visible symmetrical venous patterns.
   d. Thickened skin with enlarged pores.

5. The number and incidences of STDs are increasing dramatically among women. Women most at risk are:

   a. Young well-educated teenagers.
   b. Urban dwelling, low income women
   c. Middle-class well established women
   d. Women in the work force.

6. Major health concerns of adult women tend to be related to changes associated with aging. What is aging?

   a. A natural biologic process that affects physiologic and psychological health.
   b. A deterioration process that begins during late adulthood.
   c. The promotion and maintenance of optimal health through exercising and dieting.
   d. The devalued status of a woman in a culturally deprived area.

WOMEN'S HEALTH ACROSS THE LIFE SPAN

Matching Exercise of Critical Content

Match the definitions listed on the right with the correct terms.

_____ 1. Amenorrhea
_____ 2. Endometriosis
_____ 3. PMS
_____ 4. Dysmenorrhea
_____ 5. Fibrocystic Disease
_____ 6. Cervicitis
_____ 7. Fibroid tumors
_____ 8. TSS
_____ 9. Bacterial Vaginosis
_____ 10. PID
_____ 11. UTI

A. Palpable irregular breast tissue
B. Benign uterine growth
C. Inflammation of epithelial cells
D. Implants of tissue outside uterus
E. Cluster of cyclic symptoms
F. Absence of menstrual cycle
G. Painful menstruation
H. Bacteria in urinary tract
I. Rare multi-system disorder
J. Common vaginal infection
K. Common progression of an STD

Critical Thinking Exercise

1. Evaluate the following three adjustments of young adulthood; vocational, marital or singleness, and parenthood. Relate two problems and two satisfactions inherent in each.

2. Jennifer Azure, age 50, has come to the clinic for her annual physical. She states that she does not seem to have as much energy as she had a couple of years ago and that lately she has been having some problems seeing and hearing. Formulate a teaching plan for Ms. Azure on the aging process. Be sure to include interventions to assist her in the adjustment to the aging process.

CHAPTER 7

Fertility Management

Overview

Fertility is the capacity of our bodies to create, nurture, and sustain a fetus. For many women, adapting to their fertility will at certain times mean seeking ways to prevent or postpone pregnancy, whereas for other women fertility itself may be in question. This chapter explores these two distinct but complimentary areas of the reproductive health spectrum.

Learning Objectives

After studying the material in this chapter, the student will be able to:

- Discuss trends in contraceptive use among women in the United States.

- Define typical failure rate and discuss three factors affecting method effectiveness.

- List contraceptive methods available in the United States and discuss the effectiveness, the contraceptive action, health benefits, and side effects of each method.

- State the contraindications to oral contraceptive use and link these to the major complications that can occur with this method.

- Discuss special contraceptive needs of women after unprotected intercourse, during the postpartum period, over age 35, and if they are infected with human immunodeficiency virus.

- List and discuss at least four nursing responsibilities in counseling for contraceptive use.

- Discuss the relationship of gestational age to safety of elective abortion.

- Explain the most common causes of infertility and their treatments.

- Discuss two ethical problems related to assisted reproductive technologies.

FERTILITY MANAGEMENT

Application of Key Terms

Match the definition in column two with the key terms in column one.

1. Abstinence
2. Basal body temperature
3. Calendar method
4. Cervical cap
5. Coitus interruptus
6. Diaphragm
7. Dilation and evacuation
8. Endometrial biopsy
9. Fertility
10. Gamete intrafallopian tube transfer
11. Hysterosalpingogram
12. Intrauterine device
13. In vitro fertilization
14. Postcoital protection
15. Postcoital test
16. Primary infertility
17. Semen analysis
18. Spermicide
19. Sterilization
20. Vacuum curettage
21. Vasectomy

A. Process whereby ova are extracted surgically from a woman, fertilized in a test tube, and implanted in the uterus.

B. Inability to conceive or carry a pregnancy to viability with no previous history of pregnancy carried to live birth.

C. Diagnostic procedure in which a sample of cervical mucus is extracted within about 6 hours of sexual intercourse.

D. Abstention from sexual intercourse.

E. Procedure in which the uterine cervix is dilated and the uterine contents removed.

F. Method of male sterilization in which the vas deferens are cut and ligated to prevent sperm from entering the ejaculate.

G. Diagnostic procedure in which radiopaque dye is injected into the cervix, uterus, and fallopian tubes to determine their patency.

H. Diagnostic procedure in which a sample of endometrial tissue is obtained.

I. Agent that kills spermatozoa.

J. Temperature when body metabolism is at its lowest; used as a method to determine when ovulation occurs.

K. Small metal or plastic form placed in the uterus to prevent implantation of fertilized ovum.

L. Process rendering a person unable to produce children.

M. Method in which the products of conception are extracted from the uterus by suction.

N. Withdrawal of the penis from the vagina prior to ejaculation.

O. A method of natural family planning based upon the assumptions that ovulation occurs on day 14, sperm is viable for 72 hours, and ovum survives 24 hours.

P. The capacity of our bodies to create, nurture, and sustain the earliest lives of our children.

Q. Cup-shaped soft rubber devices that fit directly over the cervix.

R. Dome-shaped rubber cups with a flexible spring rim inserted to cover the cervix.

S. A mechanism comprised of ovarian hyperstimulation, externally mixing sperm and ovum; placement of ovocyte/sperm mixture into fallopian tube, and administering progesterone.

T. A method to determine normal sperm count, motility, morphology, pH, and viscosity of semen.

U. "Morning after" birth control.

Short Answer Exercise of Critical Content

1. Describe five characteristics of the ideal contraceptive.

   a.

   b.

   c.

   d.

   e.

2. Use the acronym "ACHES" to list the oral contraceptive danger signs.

   A.

   C.

   H.

   E.

   S.

FERTILITY MANAGEMENT

3. Use the acronym "PAINS" to list the IUD-use danger signs.

   P.

   A.

   I.

   N.

   S.

4. In the following table, compare each of the contraceptive methods in terms of advantages and disadvantages by supplying the missing information.

	Advantages	Disadvantages
Diaphragm	a.	b.
Cervical Cap	c.	d.
Sponges	e.	f.
Vaginal Pouch	g.	h.
Condoms	i.	j.
Foams, Jellies	k.	l.
Oral Contraceptives	m.	n.
Norplant	o.	p.
IUD	q.	r.
Sterilization	s.	t.

5. List and describe the four variations of natural family planning.

   a.

   b.

   c.

   d.

6. Complete the following sentences by furnishing the missing word(s).

   a. _____ is the inability to conceive or carry a pregnancy to viability with no previous history of a pregnancy carried to a live birth.

   b. _____ is the inability to conceive or carry a pregnancy to a live birth following one or more successful pregnancies.

   c. _____ refers to individuals whose life situations preclude the occurrence of conception.

7. Identify three main factors contributing to infertility in woman and include rate.

   a.

   b.

   c.

8. Identify two main factors contributing to male infertility and include rate.

   a.

   b.

FERTILITY MANAGEMENT

9. Mr. and Mrs. Cook come to the infertility clinic. They have been attempting a pregnancy for three years. Mrs. Cook had an ectopic pregnancy during a previous marriage. She also tells you that she has regular monthly periods that last 3-4 days.

   a. Identify what you think needs to be done to assess this couple for infertility and why?

   b. Plan treatment options that might be available to them and include why?

10. Complete the following chart on procedures used in the evaluation of infertility by providing the missing information.

Procedure	Parameter(s) Assessed	Description
Semen analysis	a.	b.
Sims-Huhner Test	c.	d.
BBT Chart	e.	f.
Hysterosalpingogram	g.	h.
Endometrial Biopsy	i.	j.

Multiple Choice Exercise of Critical Content

Circle the most correct answer

1. The time of ovulation may be determined by taking the basal temperature. The temperature.
   a. Drops at the time of ovulation
   b. Drops and then rises at the time of ovulation
   c. Drops, rises, and drops again at the time of ovulation.
   d. Remains constant throughout the menstrual cycle.

2. Zola appears at the abortion clinic and is confirmed to be 8 weeks pregnant. She is requesting an abortion. Legal abortions may be performed.

   a. Without a state's interference if they are doctor-approved and done within the first three months of pregnancy.

   b. Only in those states that have liberalized abortion laws.

   c. Only to preserve the woman's health.

   d. During the last trimester of pregnancy, and they are subject only to the consent of the male and female involved.

3. After Zola's abortion, she asks questions about birth control methods. If correctly used, which of the following methods of birth control provides virtually 100% effectiveness?

   a. Intrauterine devices.

   b. Diaphragm

   c. Oral contraceptives

   d. Coitus interruptus

4. Zola questions the method of obtaining a birth control method. She requires a cheap, easy to obtain method. Which of the following contraceptives requires consultation with a physician?

   a. Coitus interruptus

   b. Vaginal foams

   c. Diaphragm

   d. Condom

5. Zola is educated about the methods of birth control. You remind her that the use of effective birth control methods facilitates:

   a. Population growth control

   b. Reduced anxiety over unwanted pregnancy

   c. Family planning

   d. All of the above

6. Helen has used an oral contraceptive since the birth of her last child. She has not been happy with the choice because of the need to take the pills regularly. Although the method by which oral contraceptives prevent pregnancy is not entirely clear, the general assumption is that they do so by:

   a. Preventing implantation

   b. Suppressing ovulation

   c. Altering the receptivity of the endometrium

   d. Destroying the sperm

FERTILITY MANAGEMENT

7. Many of Helen's friends use the IUD to prevent pregnancy. She asks about the device, its effectiveness, and its safety. The IUD is thought to prevent pregnancy by:
   a. Preventing ovulation
   b. Interfering with implantation
   c. Destroying the sperm
   d. Disrupting function of fallopian tubes

8. Helen and Peter are considering vasectomy as a method of contraception. Vasectomy is accomplished by:
   a. Excising the testicles
   b. Excising the prostate
   c. Bilateral ligation of the vas deferens
   d. A major surgical procedure

9. Peter wants to know if he will be immediately and permanently sterile after the vasectomy. Which of the following statements regarding the procedure are true?
   a. Sperm may be present up to 8 weeks after the procedure
   b. The procedure is completely nonreversible
   c. The male is sperm-free immediately after the procedure
   d. Vasectomy is not 100% effective as a birth control method

10. Jennifer had a miscarriage 2 years ago. She and her partner have been trying to conceive a child for the past 18 months. Which of the following terms best describes her condition?
    a. Normal variation
    b. Primary infertility
    c. Secondary infertility
    d. Sterility

11. Jennifer is taught to check her mucus for signs of ovulation. The term spinnbarkheit refers to:
    a. The changes in cervical mucus that occur throughout the ovulatory cycle
    b. The distinct fern pattern of the cervical mucus at the time of ovulation
    c. The increased elasticity of the cervical mucus at the time of ovulation
    d. The midcycle or ovulatory pain some women experience

12. Jennifer's partner is found to have a sperm count of 53 million/mL. This indicates he has:
    a. A borderline sperm count
    b. A normal sperm count
    c. To be considered infertile
    d. To be considered sterile

UNIT II: DYNAMICS OF HUMAN REPRODUCTION

Matching Exercise of Critical Content

Match the following. Match the definitions in column B with the reproductive technologies in column A. Some answers may be used more than once. Some blanks have more than one answer.

_____ 1. IVF
_____ 2. GIFT
_____ 3. IVF with donor egg and gestational carrier

A. Pregnancy and birth rate success is better
B. Ovarian hyperstimulation
C. Surrogate
D. Oocytes transferred to a culture
E. Washed sperm mixed with oocytes
F. 3-4 embryos placed in uterus
G. Oocyte/sperm mixture placed at end of fallopian tube
H. Expensive

True and False Exercise of Critical Content

The following statements require you to assess whether they are true or false. Circle the correct response (true or false). If the statements is false, rewrite it so that it is correct.

1. The legal system has determined that the rights of the gestational mother are superior to the rights of the genetic mother. (True/False)

2. Serious emotional stresses are created in response to high reproductive technology treatment. (True/False).

3. Nurses working with individuals with infertility should reassure the couple that the procedure is simple. (True/False).

4. During a year of diagnosis and treatment, women increased their sense of mastery over life, self-esteem, and support from partners. (True/False).

FERTILITY MANAGEMENT

5. The high cost of artificial reproductive technology approximates the high costs of intensive care units. (True/False).

6. A thorough evaluation and conventional treatment for ovarian drug treatment is estimated at $9000 per woman in 1992 and is successful only about 30% of the time. (True/False)

Critical Thinking Exercises

1. You have been asked to prepare a discussion class about the different types of contraceptives. Design a chart that you could use to present the different types of contraceptives including the mechanism(s) of action, safety, and benefits.

2. Roselinda approaches you after visiting a reproductive specialist. She is very emotional and asks you what she should do. Evaluate what she has been told, apprise her of the different tests that may be conducted and assist her in formulating questions to ask the reproductive specialist.

UNIT III: ADAPTATION IN THE PRENATAL PERIOD

CHAPTER 8

Individual and Family Adaptation to Pregnancy

Overview

Pregnancy and childbirth are events that touch nearly every aspect of the human experience: biological, psychological, social, and cultural. Variations in age, health, socioeconomic status, and cultural background of the woman and her family will influence health care needs. This chapter discusses the definition, structure, and function of families and how they necessitate adaptations. Major social, cultural, and psychological patterns describe how people adapt to the childbearing experience. The study of these patterns spans several disciplines, including sociology, anthropology, and psychology.

Learning Objectives

After studying the material in this chapter, the student will be able to:

- Identify major social factors that influence decisions about childbearing.

- Describe how birth practices may vary across cultures.

- Discuss nursing strategies for assessing cultural variations in birth practices.

- Explain basic functions and developmental tasks of the childbearing family.

- Describe the crisis potential of pregnancy and explain why family crises may occur during pregnancy and how they can be prevented.

- List maternal and paternal tasks during pregnancy and discuss their significance for healthy individual and family adaptation.

- Identify common maternal and paternal responses to pregnancy and suggest nursing interventions.

INDIVIDUAL AND FAMILY ADAPTATION TO PREGNANCY

Application of Key Terms

Match the definitions in column two with the key terms in column one.

_____ 1. Acculturation
_____ 2. Attachment
_____ 3. Cognitive processes
_____ 4. Couvade syndrome
_____ 5. Cultural relativism
_____ 6. Developmental task
_____ 7. Ethnocentrism
_____ 8. Maturational crisis
_____ 9. Situational crisis

A. Practice of judging a group or its traits by its own or similar standards.

B. Belief in the natural superiority of the group to which one belongs; tendency to judge a group by standards appropriate to another group.

C. Affiliative tie formed after a period of mutual stimulation and response.

D. Step, stage, or phase in the process of growth that is sequential and prerequisite to further growth.

E. Beliefs and practices are modified or dropped in favor of practices of the dominant culture.

F. A constellation of symptoms much like those the pregnant woman experiences.

G. Arising from a change in events or life circumstances.

H. Processes involved in perceiving, interpreting, organizing, storing, retrieving, coordinating, and using stimuli received from the internal and external environment.

I. Arising from internal changes in the individual or family, associated with normal growth and development.

Short Answer Exercise of Critical Content

1. Joe and Susi are expecting their first child. Joe has been working as many extra shifts as possible. At home he has been doing more of the house work and is painting the nursery. Susi has been visiting garage sales every weekend to find baby furniture and clothing. Sometimes her mother (Elaine) accompanies Susi to the sales. They have fun together and share a lot about Elaine's experiences with pregnancy. Joe and Susi have been able to openly share their fears, expectations, and feelings with each other. What developmental tasks are Susi and Joe working on?

2. Joe and Susi realize there will be many changes in their relationship and in their roles as they prepare for parenthood. List and define five maternal tasks Susi will need to accomplish during her pregnancy.

   a.

   b.

   c.

   d.

   e.

3. How do Susi's tasks compare with the tasks Joe needs to accomplish during pregnancy?

4. Some nurses view psychosocial and cultural aspects of maternity nursing as much less important than the clinical or physical aspects, yet they are very important to client care. Identify at least five psychosocial/cultural factors that affect decisions to become pregnant.

   a.

   b.

   c.

   d.

   e.

INDIVIDUAL AND FAMILY ADAPTATION TO PREGNANCY

5. Identify at least five psychosocial/cultural assessments the nurse should make when working with a pregnant client.

   a.

   b.

   c.

   d.

   e.

6. The nurse in labor and delivery has just been notified that a Vietnamese woman, age 30, is to be admitted for induction of post-term labor. When she arrives at the hospital, she is alone except for a two year old child. She does not speak any English but smiles pleasantly at the nurse and frequently nods yes to any question or statement directed toward her. What will be the nurse's first priority?

7. How might the nurse begin to obtain basic assessment data and routine laboratory specimens?

Multiple Choice Exercises of Critical Content

Circle the most correct answer

1. Maslow's hierarchy of needs suggests that basic physiologic needs must be met before the individual can reach his or her fullest potential. An example of a physiological need being met would be:
   a. The need to be well thought of by oneself as well as by others.
   b. Obtaining prenatal care during the first trimester.
   c. Building an extra room for the baby onto a small house.
   d. Drinking eight glasses of water a day and following a well balanced diet.

2. A family is the fundamental unit of all human societies. A currently accepted definition of family as used by social scientists might include:

   a. A social system made up of two or more interdependent persons.
   b. A group of interacting and interdependent personalities.
   c. A group related by blood, marriage, or adoption.
   d. All of the above are currently accepted definitions.

3. Pregnancy has been defined as a crisis. Successful resolution of a crisis depends upon:

   a. The ability to remain isolated and not use other resources.
   b. The continuation of the crisis, anxiety, and stress.
   c. The range of coping patterns available.
   d. How unrealistically the situation is perceived.

4. Mary Lou is in her third trimester and has begun to sing and talk to the fetus. Mary Lou is probably exhibiting signs of:

   a. Mental illness.
   b. Delusions.
   c. Attachment.
   d. Crisis.

5. Mary Lou's husband Steven has begun to put on weight. This could possibly be a sign of:

   a. Culturalism syndrome.
   b. Couvade syndrome.
   c. Maturational crisis.
   d. Attachment.

6. Janelle is pregnant for the second time. Her son, Steven, has just turned 2 years old. She ask you what she should do to help him get ready for the expected birth. Your answer might include which of the following:

   a. If Steven's sleeping arrangements are to be changed, these changes should be done well before Janelle goes into labor.
   b. Steven will probably resent Janelle's physical limitations, such as her inability to lift, hold, or rough house with him.
   c. She should encourage Steven to plan an elaborate welcome for the newborn and help with the newborn's care.
   d. Steven will probably not understand any explanations about the arrival of a new brother or sister so Janelle should do nothing.

INDIVIDUAL AND FAMILY ADAPTATION TO PREGNANCY

Matching Content of Critical Content

Match the definitions for different types of families in column two with the terms in column one.

Terms	Definitions
____ 1. Extended family	A. Adults who have remarried and are raising children from the previous marriage.
____ 2. Nuclear dyad	B. An adult head-of-household with one or more dependent children.
____ 3. Nuclear family	C. Male-female couples living without children in a single family residence.
____ 4. Blended family	D. Parents and dependent children living in a single family residence away from family of origin.
____ 5. Single-parent family	E. Two or more households of any type that look to each other for support and frequent interaction.

Match the variations in birth practices listed in column two with the cultural/ethnic group listed in column one.

Group	Variation
____ 1. Asian American	A. Preserving the umbilical cord and keeping it in the home.
____ 2. Japanese	B. Belief that many children assure parents of a high place in heaven.
____ 3. African American	C. Extended family, particularly woman's mother, is a major source of support.
____ 4. Mormon	D. Withholding food and drink during labor.
____ 5. Mexican American	E. Politeness and deference to authority; true feelings hidden.
____ 6. Southeastern Asian American	F. Woman and fetus are vulnerable to outside bad influences.
____ 7. European American	G. Woman is expected to stay close to infant and satisfy its needs immediately.
____ 8. Arab American	H. Husband is involved in all aspects of wife's care.

True and False Exercise of Critical Content

The following statements require you to assess whether or not they are true or false. If the statement is false, rewrite it so that it is correct.

1. A major goal of perinatal nursing care is to help families make the healthiest adjustment to the normal stresses of the childbearing year. (True/False).

2. An exploratory study of 26 couples was conducted to examine what parents know about their fetus. The findings indicated that these couples were unaware of the fetus. (True/False).

3. Concepts of reproductive decisions are mainly secretive and very individualized. (True/False).

4. Individual and family adaptation to pregnancy is a complex process that requires extensive psychological, physical, and social adjustments over a fairly brief period of time. (True/False).

5. Pregnancy is not a time of increased vulnerability to crisis. (True/False).

Critical Thinking Exercises

1. Decide what the major ethnic cultures are in the city/community where you live: Indicate the dominant religions. Contrast these dominant groups with the other areas of your state and the United States as a whole. Identify the agencies/resources where you obtained this information. Evaluate the hospitals/agencies in your community in regard to their tendency to work more with one particular sub-cultural or ethnic group. Why?

2. Analyze what you believe is the ideal time to bear one's first child. Why? Formulate criteria you believe is important for readiness to have children. Compare your criteria with your classmates and at least one client/family you have worked with in a clinical setting.

3. Develop a list of questions to assess a father's adaptation to pregnancy. Plan an interview with a man whose wife is pregnant for the first time. Evaluate how well he is accomplishing the paternal tasks of pregnancy. Generate ways you could help him adapt to the pregnancy and parenthood. Write your findings and insights in a clinical paper and contrast your results with those of classmates.

CHAPTER 9

Adolescent Childbearing and Parenting

Overview

Adolescent sexual activity and adolescent pregnancy are major health problems in the United States and Canada. One million American adolescent pregnancies result in approximately 500,000 births and 400,000 induced abortions each year. Teen pregnancy rates in the United States have leveled off and declined minimally since 1976; however, the incidence of childbirth and abortion among adolescents younger than 15 years continue to climb. This chapter provides an overview of the complex subject of adolescent childbearing and parenting.

Learning Objectives

After studying the material in this chapter, the student will be able to:

- Describe the incidence of adolescent pregnancy and parenting.
- Discuss the developmental tasks of adolescence.
- Identify factors that contribute to high rates of adolescent pregnancy and parenting.
- Describe the implication of pregnancy and parenting for adolescents and their society.
- Relate poverty and limited life options to the cycle of adolescent pregnancy and parenting.
- Discuss nursing implications related to adolescent childbearing.

Application to Key Terms

Match the definitions in column two with the key terms in column one.

_____ 1. Biological maturation
_____ 2. Culture of poverty
_____ 3. Developmental tasks
_____ 4. Life options
_____ 5. Narcissism
_____ 6. Risk behaviors

A. Step, stage, or phase in the process of growth that is sequential and prerequisite to further growth.

B. Undue dwelling on one's own self or attainments.

C. Growth and development of primary and secondary sexual characteristics and the physiologic capacity to initiate pregnancy.

D. Pessimistic attitudes about opportunities for educational and vocational advancement.

E. A society characterized by low income, poor housing, poor health behaviors, and poor education.

F. An action that exposes one to possible loss or injury.

UNIT III: ADAPTATION IN THE PRENATAL PERIOD

Short Answer Exercise of Critical Content

1. Using the following chart, identify characteristics of the three adolescent stages as theorized by Holt and Johnson (1991).

Early Adolescent

a. Growth Rate	
b. Body Image	
c. Reference Group	
d. Cognitive Operations	
e. Family Relations	
f. Sexuality	

Middle Adolescence

g. Growth Rate	
h. Body Image	
i. Reference Group	
j. Cognitive Operations	
k. Family Relations	
l. Sexuality	

Late Adolescence

m. Growth Rate	
n. Body Image	
o. Reference Group	
p. Cognitive Operations	
q. Family Relations	
r. Sexuality	

ADOLESCENT CHILDBEARING AND PARENTING

2. List three reasons an adolescent might become pregnant.

   a.

   b.

   c.

3. Identify two major physiologic adaptation problems that are significant for pregnant adolescents.

   a.

   b.

4. Identify three physical health problems that are associated with adolescent pregnancy.

   a.

   b.

   c.

5. Analyze how socioeconomic and ethnic factor are indicators of risk.

Multiple Choice Exercise of Critical Content

Circle the most correct answer.

1. Adolescents who maintain their pregnancies and choose to parent cite a variety of factors affecting their decision. Such a factor might include:
   a. Enough money saved to establish a modest home for self and baby.
   b. An unsuccessful career at school and expectation that pregnancy signals adulthood.
   c. No plans to dropout of school because peers will care for baby.
   d. African Americans are more likely to leave school than Hispanic Americans.

2. Denice, a 14 year old African American, comes to the pregnancy crisis center for a pregnancy test. The test is positive and Denice appears very nonchalent about the news. Your response might be based upon the knowledge that:

   a. Denice's sexual identity is firmly established and her mental functioning is stable.

   b. Denice probably uses peers to share experiences, to avoid social isolation, and to try out adult roles.

   c. Denice uses concrete operational thinking that focuses on the present and is egocentric in nature.

   d. Denice may overestimate her power to influence events and believes this pregnancy was an act of fate.

3. You know that Denice's chances of becoming a parent again within 2 years are great because of:

   a. Her use of drugs.

   b. Her young age.

   c. Her good coping behavior.

   d. Her increased self-esteem.

4. The 17 year-old father of Denice's baby is at high risk for:

   a. High school dropout.

   b. Unemployment.

   c. Questioning his paternity.

   d. All of the above

5. An appropriate Nursing diagnosis for Denice might be:

   a. Altered family process related to adolescent pregnancy.

   b. Altered nutrition: more than body requirements related to lack of knowledge about nutritional needs.

   c. Increased self-esteem related to family acceptance and support.

   d. Social acceptance related to the reactions of peers and family to pregnancy.

ADOLESCENT CHILDBEARING AND PARENTING

Matching Exercise of Critical Content

Match the following. Some answers may be used more than once. Some blanks have more than one answer.

_____	1. Shortened Education	A.	Adolescent Woman
_____	2. Decreased Vocational Opportunities	B.	Adolescent Male
_____	3. Early Marriage		
_____	4. Single Parenthood		
_____	5. Repeat Pregnancies		
_____	6. Difficult Adapting to Parenting		

True and False Exercise of Critical Content

The following statements require you to assess whether or not they are true or false. If the statement is false, rewrite it so that it is correct.

1. Newborns of adolescent mothers are at higher risk for prematurity and low birth weight with concomitant increases in neonatal mortality and morbidity. (True/False).

2. Children of adolescent parents show no differences in attentive behavior or verbal interaction than children of nonadolescent parents. (True/False).

3. A study of African American single-parent families found that preschoolers were substantially more likely to score lower on readiness for school testing when the mother was single, a school dropout, and on welfare. (True/False).

4. Adolescent childbearing and parenting have profound effects on the health of the adolescent but does not appear to effect their children, their families, or society in general. (True/False).

5. Nurses need not concern themselves with the problem of teen pregnancy. (True/False).

Critical Thinking Exercises

1. You and four classmates have volunteered to participate in a high school discussion about pregnancy, abortion, and contraceptives. The coordinator of the program will begin the program by comparing present trends in sexuality with those of former years. It is essential that you present accurate information to the students. Create a plan and generate a list of topics.

2. Assume that your 13 year old daughter, Rose, tells you that she has missed three menstrual periods. Evaluate your response and decide what steps need to be taken.

3. Rose is pregnant and decides to have an abortion. At the follow-up visit, the office nurse shows Rose various contraceptives and lets her handle them. She encourages Rose to make another appointment soon to initiate a form of contraception before engaging in sex. Explain what the nurses motivation is for doing this.

CHAPTER 10

Childbearing and Parenting After Age 35

Overview

First-time pregnancy and parenthood for women over age 35 is increasing. Advances in reproductive technology have even made it possible for women in their early fifties to consider pregnancy. In addition, women who have previously given birth may experience repeat pregnancies beyond age 35. For some women, a late pregnancy represents a planned event to add a final member to the family unit. For others, the pregnancy is unplanned or unexpected. The nurse must be knowledgeable about the unique physical risk of later childbearing. This chapter discusses reasons for delayed childbearing and repeat pregnancy after age 35 and describes the medical and obstetric risks for the woman, fetus, and neonate.

Learning Objectives

After studying the material in this chapter, the student will be able to:

- Describe trends in childbearing for women over age 35 in the United States.
- Discuss the importance of preconception counseling for women planning pregnancy after the age of 35.
- Discuss the impact of aging on reproductive functioning and fertility in women.
- Describe how repeat pregnancy for the older multiparous woman differs from a first pregnancy for the woman over age 35.
- Identify major physiologic complications of pregnancy that are more common with advancing age.
- Discuss how the developmental tasks of pregnancy may differ for both the older primigravida and multigravida.
- List major intrapartum complications for the woman who delays childbearing beyond age 35.
- Describe how advancing age influences postpartum adjustment and maternal role attainment.
- Develop a nursing care plan for the woman over age 35 who is pregnant for the first time.

Application of Key Terms

Match the definitions in column two with the key terms in column one.

____ 1. Advanced maternal age
____ 2. Anovulatory cycle
____ 3. Dystocia
____ 4. Fertility
____ 5. Multigravida
____ 6. Multipara
____ 7. Nulligravida
____ 8. Nullipara

A. Woman who is pregnant and has been pregnant before.
B. Difficult labor resulting from fetal or maternal causes.
C. Woman who has never carried a pregnancy to the stage of viability.
D. Menstrual cycle in which menstrual flow was not preceded by discharge of an ovum.
E. Woman who is not now and never has been pregnant.
F. Woman who has completed two or more pregnancies to the stage of viability.
G. Delayed pregnancy or repeat pregnancy after age 35.
H. The capacity of one's body to create, nurture, and sustain the earliest lives of children.

Short Answer Exercise of Critical Content

1. List three special concerns of an older expectant couple.

   a.

   b.

   c.

2. Identify two factors influencing the decision to become a parent after age 35.

   a.

   b.

3. What steps can a nurse take to assist the older mother adjust to pregnancy, labor, delivery, and postpartum.

CHILDBEARING AND PARENTING AFTER AGE 35

Multiple Choice Exercise of Critical Content

Circle the most correct answer.

1. Martha, a 37 year-old married executive is told her pregnancy test is positive. Martha is very excited about this first pregnancy. You realize that Martha is at increased risk for:
   a. No complications with this pregnancy.
   b. Spontaneous abortion with this pregnancy.
   c. Financial constraints due to inadequate insurance.
   d. Lack of knowledge regarding child care due to low educational preparation.

2. Martha's pregnancy is progressing and at 20 weeks appears in labor and delivery with contractions. A bolus of I.V. fluids and bed rest results in diminishing the contractions. The health care provider will probably advise Martha to:
   a. Quit work immediately and remain on strict bed rest.
   b. Continue as she is, working 60 hours a week.
   c. Cut back work to no more than 40 hours per week, force fluids, and rest more frequently.
   d. Go on a strict salt free diet, do simple exercises, and increase diet drinks.

3. Martha successfully completes her pregnancy and delivers a 7 lb, 8 oz baby boy. Her husband was present at the delivery and displays ability to care for the infant following delivery. You enter Martha's room to find her dictating to her husband every step he should do to change the diaper. A possible nursing diagnoses would be which of the following:
   a. Knowledge deficit related to inability to learn routine care.
   b. Body image disturbance related to pregnancy.
   c. Altered family processes related to change in family roles and gain of family member.
   d. Ineffective individual coping related to change in work role.

4. Your hospital has a follow-up program that provides a home visit within the first 72 hours after delivery and a telephone call after 6 days. You refer Martha to this program because:
   a. She will probably become an abusive mother and must be taught proper care.
   b. She will need someone to stay with the baby so she can go back to work.
   c. She cannot trust her husband to provide any care for the new baby.
   d. Discharge is a difficult time and the support will assist with the transition.

True and False Exercise of Critical Content

The following statements require you to assess whether or not they are true or false. If the statement is false, rewrite it so that it is correct.

1. The number of women giving birth after age 35 is increasing because of the sudden increase in population growth after World War II. (True/False).

2. For most women, repeat pregnancy after age 35 is a planned event. (True/False).

3. Many women age 35 or older delay pregnancy because of choice rather than because of infertility problems. (True/False).

4. The incidence of spontaneous abortion rate is approximately 10% at age 20; 18% by the late thirties and 34% in the mid forties. (True/False).

5. Healthy older women without previous medical or obstetric complications are still more likely to experience both prenatal and intrapartum problems. (True/False).

6. Statistics indicate that the older pregnant woman has probably been employed, at least part-time, for most of her adult life. (True/False).

7. Some evidence indicates that men in their thirties may feel very insecure in their identity and in the couple relationship, and these factors may delay the older first-time father's achievement of the paternal role. (True/False).

8. The greatest challenge for nurses may be nursing care of the older multiparous woman whose unplanned conception is complicated by poverty. (True/False).

Critical Thinking Exercises

1. Marla, a 38 year old primigravida, comes to you for assistance in preparing for her upcoming delivery. Marla is 30 weeks pregnant. Develop a plan to prepare her for the up coming delivery and the transition to motherhood. Prepare a list of potential resources.

2. Analyze the reasons an older first-time mother would be more likely to verbalize disappointment with her birth experience. Structure a plan to optimize the birth experience for the older primigravida when complications arise during labor.

CHAPTER 11

Physiologic Adaptations in Pregnancy

Overview

The period from conception to delivery is approximately 40 weeks long. During these weeks the woman's body undergoes complex physiologic changes of such magnitude that many are still not well understood. Every system in the woman's body adapts to the demands of the growing fetus. This chapter discusses the changes produced by pregnancy in the structure and function of the various systems and organs of the body.

Learning Objectives

After studying the material in this chapter, the student will be able to:

- Describe the major physiologic adaptations that occur during pregnancy and recognize their causes.

- Describe the altered physiology of pregnancy to the woman as appropriate.

- Demonstrate an understanding of physiologic adaptations and their effects on the pregnant woman.

- Discuss the normal adaptation of the reproductive organs in pregnancy.

- Identify changes in the endocrine function during pregnancy.

- Explain the actions of the steroid hormones progesterone and estrogen in pregnancy.

Application of Key Terms

Match the definitions in column two with the key terms in column one.

____ 1. Collagenous
____ 2. Diaphoretic
____ 3. Essential hypertension
____ 4. Glomerular filtration rate
____ 5. Glucocorticoids
____ 6. Glucogenesis
____ 7. Homeostasis
____ 8. Hygroscopic
____ 9. Hyperemia
____ 10. Hyperplasia
____ 11. Hypertrophy
____ 12. Hyperventilation
____ 13. Hypervolemia
____ 14. Interstitial
____ 15. Ketones
____ 16. Metabolite
____ 17. Neurohumoral
____ 18. Nocturia
____ 19. Precursor
____ 20. Shunt
____ 21. Sinusoids
____ 22. Syncytiotrophoblasts

A. State of equilibrium in the internal environment of the body that is naturally maintained by adaptive body responses.

B. Passage that diverts flow from one main route to another.

C. Formation of glucose in the liver from sources that are not carbohydrates, such as fatty or amino acids.

D. Increased blood flow to a part as evidenced by redness of the skin.

E. End products of fat metabolism.

F. Profuse perspiration.

G. Any product of metabolism.

H. Outer layer of cells covering the chorionic villi of the placenta that is in contact with the maternal blood.

I. Pertaining to fibrous protein found in connective tissue, such as bone, ligaments, and cartilage.

J. Blood pressure higher than normal for age that develops in the absence of kidney disease.

K. Pertaining to a substance that readily absorbs moisture.

L. Excessive urination during the night.

M. Increase in size of an organ or structure not resulting from an increase in the number of cells.

N. Small blood vessels found in the liver, spleen, and adrenal glands.

O. Substance that precedes the production of another substance.

P. Amount of plasma filtered by the glomeruli of both kidneys per minute.

Q. Excessive proliferation of normal cell substances in the normal arrangement of a structure or organ.

R. Increased, forced respiration that may induce dizziness or fainting.

S. Referring to spaces within a tissue or organ.

T. Adrenal hormones that are active in protecting against stress and also affect protein and carbohydrate metabolism.

U. Diminished blood volume.

V. Chemicals liberated at nerve endings that excite adjacent structures.

PHYSIOLOGIC ADAPTATIONS IN PREGNANCY

Short Answer Exercise of Critical Content

1. In formulating a prenatal teaching plan identify information that should be included to prepare the pregnant woman for physical changes in each of the following structures.

    a. Uterus

    b. Breasts

    c. Skin

    d. Vagina

    e. Gastrointestinal tract.

2. Explain changes in the cardiovascular system as a result of pregnancy.

    a. Heart

    b. Blood volume

    c. Cardiac output

    d. Heart rate

    e. Stroke volume

    f. Blood pressure

Multiple Choice Exercise of Critical Content

Circle the most correct answer.

1. At the end of the first trimester of pregnancy, there is:
   a. An increase in blood volume.
   b. A decrease in the stroke volume of the heart.
   c. An increase in the diastolic blood pressure.
   d. A decrease in total blood volume.

2. The substance responsible for a positive reactions to a pregnancy test is:
   a. Estrogen.
   b. Progesterone.
   c. Chorionic Gonadotropin.
   d. Prolactin.

3. Zoe reports that she is 8 weeks pregnant and that she has been nauseated all day for the past four days. You know this is probably due to:
   a. Significant liver changes that accompany pregnancy.
   b. Sluggish and somewhat impaired function.
   c. Eating coal, clay, laundry starch or other inappropriate substances.
   d. Fluid pooling in the lower extremities and causing lower renal congestion.

4. Harrideen reports that her mother-in-law believes that rubbing goose grease on her stretch marks will make them go away. You could inform her that:
   a. She should continue this process every day.
   b. She is gaining too much weight and that is why she has numerous striae.
   c. She should expose her abdomen to the sunshine for at least one hour every day.
   d. After delivery striae recede to silverish marks but never fully go away.

PHYSIOLOGIC ADAPTATIONS IN PREGNANCY

Matching Exercise of Critical Content

Match the hormone with the corresponding effects associated with pregnancy. All hormones in the list are not used.

Hormonal Effects of Pregnancy

___ 1. Softens pubic joints
___ 2. Enhances absorption of nutrients
___ 3. Milk let-down reflex initiated
___ 4. Uterine growth promoted
___ 5. Effects unknown
___ 6. Calcium metabolism altered
___ 7. Fatty acid metabolism increased
___ 8. Corpus luteum preserved

Hormone

A. Estrogen
B. Glucocorticoid
C. Human Chorionic Gonadotropin (HCG)
D. Human Placental Lactogen (HPL)
E. Oxytocin
F. Parathyroid Hormone
G. Prostaglandin
H. Relaxin
I. Thyroxine

Critical Thinking Exercise

1. Formulate a teaching plan to provide anticipatory guidance in assisting the prenatal client to adapt to the physical changes of pregnancy. Include all systems and explain ways to overcome some of the symptoms.

2. Analyze a prenatal record of a pregnant woman. Evaluate weight gain pattern, hemoglobin and hematocrit levels, fundal height measurements and evidence of fluid retention during each month of gestation. Compare your findings with the normal anticipated changes.

CHAPTER 12

The Genetic Code and Fetal Development

Overview

Environmental and genetic factors affect health before conception and during the prenatal period. It is useful to understand the processes of transfer of genetic information from parents to children, the progression of normal embryonic and fetal development, and the sensitive periods when fetal damage is most likely to occur. This chapter includes an overview of the genetic code, normal fetal development, and the major genetic causes of abnormal fetal development.

Learning Objectives

After studying the material in this chapter, the student will be able to:

- Describe the significant events in fetal development.
- Explain how genes are transmitted in families.
- List the major categories of genetic disorders.
- Identify factors that can cause genetic disorders.
- Explain how risk for genetic disorders is assessed.
- Identify groups of women and men who may need referral for genetic counseling and evaluation.

THE GENETIC CODE AND FETAL DEVELOPMENT

Application of Key Terms

Match the definitions in column two with the key terms in column one.

_____ 1. Autosome
_____ 2. Chromosome
_____ 3. Deoxyribonucleic acid
_____ 4. Gene
_____ 5. Karyotype
_____ 6. Meiosis
_____ 7. Mitosis
_____ 8. Monosomy
_____ 9. Pedigree
_____ 10. Sex chromosome
_____ 11. Teratogen
_____ 12. Trisomy
_____ 13. Zygote

A. Cell produced by union of the sperm and egg.
B. Chromosomal makeup of the nucleus of a human cell.
C. Chromosome responsible for sex determination.
D. Any of the 22 ordinary paired chromosomes.
E. Cell division occurring in germ cells and leading to the production of gametes containing half the usual number of chromosomes.
F. One of several microscopic rod-shaped bodies within the nucleus of a dividing cell that contain the hereditary material (genes) of the organism.
G. Chromosome disorder in which three copies of homologous chromosomes are present rather than two.
H. The smallest unit of heredity.
I. Cell division leading to the production of two daughter cells.
J. Substance that causes abnormal development of embryonic structures.
K. Chromosome disorder in which one chromosome of a pair is missing.
L. A macromolecule composed of three types of chemical units.
M. A diagrammatic representation of the family history.

Short Answer Exercise of Critical Content

1. The following are the results of chromosome studies. Beside each, write out what each karyotype denotes.

    a. 46, XX
    b. 45, XO
    c. 46, XY
    d. 47, XY + 13
    e. 47, XXY
    f. 46, XX 5p-
    g. 47, XX + 21

2. List four aspects of a client's history that may lead to an increased risk of having a child with a genetic disorder.

   a.

   b.

   c.

   d.

3. Identify five ways fetal circulation differs from that of the newborn and infant.

   a.

   b.

   c.

   d.

   e.

4. Define the following terms.

   a. Autosomal dominant

   b. Autosomal recessive

   c. X-linked dominant

   d. X-linked recessive

THE GENETIC CODE AND FETAL DEVELOPMENT

5. You are teaching a prenatal class and Ms. Bliss asks you why she should avoid teratogenic substances. Explain to her and the class the potentially harmful effects of teratogenic substances.

Multiple Choice Exercise of Critical Content

Circle the most correct answer.

1. Julie is a carrier of the X-linked disorder hemophilia. Identify the statistical probability that any boys she gives birth to will have hemophilia:
    a. 25%.
    b. 50%.
    c. 75%.
    d. 100%.

2. Jonetta, an African American primigravida, has just been diagnosed with sickle cell anemia. Sickle cell anemia is an example of a/an:
    a. Autosomal, dominant, inherited disorder.
    b. Autosomal, recessive, inherited disorder.
    c. Multifactorial, inherited disorder.
    d. X-linked, recessive, inherited disorder.

3. Bill and Joan ask about the way heredity and environment may affect their baby. The nurse responds that heredity refers to:
    a. Conditions in the womb such as blood supply and drugs that the mother takes.
    b. Psychologic factors such as love and cultural factors such as social class.
    c. Nutritional status of mother and presence of disease processes.
    d. Heredity is determined only at the moment of conception.

4. The nurse goes on to tell Bill and Joan that most physical traits are the result of the interaction of:
    a. One pair of genes.
    b. All body systems.
    c. 10 pairs of genes.
    d. Many pairs of genes

UNIT III: ADAPTATION IN THE PRENATAL PERIOD

5. Specific characteristics passed from parents to their offspring are transmitted by:
   a. Genes.
   b. Chromosomes.
   c. Hormones.
   d. Oogenesis.

6. Fertilization of the ovum by the sperm usually occurs:
   a. In the pelvic cavity.
   b. In the fundal section of the uterus.
   c. In the distal one-third of the fallopian tube.
   d. In the corpus luteum.

7. During an ultrasonic examination the health care provider can detect the fetal heartbeat as early as the _____ of gestation.
   a. Fifth week.
   b. Ninth week.
   c. Third week.
   d. Twelfth week.

8. The health care provider will usually check for fetal heart tones with the fetoscope. The fetal heartbeat can be heard with the fetoscope by which week of gestation?
   a. Sixth.
   b. Twelfth.
   c. Twentieth.
   d. Ninth.

THE GENETIC CODE AND FETAL DEVELOPMENT

Matching Exercise of Critical Content

Match the following time frames (gestational period) during the fetal period with the appropriate descriptor.

Gestational Period	Description
____ 1. 9-12 weeks	A. The fetus will probably survive if born; however, lungs are immature.
____ 2. 13-16 weeks	B. Skin remains red and wrinkled and the fetus is covered with vernix; the lungs are beginning to produce surfactant.
____ 3. 17-20 weeks	
____ 4. 21-23 weeks	C. Both testes have descended into the scrotum; the fetus is fully developed.
____ 5. 24-27 weeks	
____ 6. 28-31 weeks	D. Lanugo has disappeared from its face but remains on its head; the vernix has become thick and protective.
____ 7. 32-36 weeks	E. For the first time, the kidneys secrete urine and the fetus begins to swallow amniotic fluid.
____ 8. 37-39 weeks	
____ 9. 40 weeks	F. Eyelids open for the first time; the fetus appears red in color due to the absence of subcutaneous fat.
	G. At the beginning of this period the male and female external genitalia appear similar; by the end of the period the genitalia are distinguishable.
	H. Brown fat is formed and the sebaceous glands secrete sebum forming vernix caseosa.
	I. There is an increase in the accumulation of subcutaneous fat and the testicles descend into the scrotum of the male.

Hereditary disorders are classified into three main etiological categories. Classify each of the following by writing the letter of the corresponding etiological category in front of the disorder.

____ 1. Trisomy 13

____ 2. Achondroplasia

____ 3. Turner syndrome

____ 4. Pyloric stenosis

____ 5. Mosaic down syndrome

____ 6. Cri du chat

____ 7. Neural tube defect

____ 8. Phenylketonuria

____ 9. Duchenne muscular dystropy

A. Chromosome disorder.

B. Single gene disorder.

C. Multifactorial disorder.

Critical Thinking Exercise

1. Prepare a list of all the over-the-counter medications that might be consumed during a pregnancy, such as cold preparations, laxatives, diuretics, aspirin, and sinus medications. Compare your list with your classmates. Determine how easy it would be to take a number of items early in a pregnancy, out of habit, without considering the neonatal outcome. Discuss the parental guilt that may develop when parents are confronted with a neonate with a birth defect.

2. Develop a genetic screening questionnaire for use in taking a genetic history. Plan the questionnaire to include a list of specific questions about genetic diseases. Remember to provide clear instructions for answering your questionnaire. Structure the questionnaire by keeping the words as appropriate to the reading level of the target population as possible.

CHAPTER 13

Nursing Assessment of the Pregnant Woman

Overview

The value of prenatal care provided in the outpatient setting cannot be overstated. At no other time in life does a healthy woman need health care with such regularity. Prenatal care does not guarantee a normal neonate, but it can identify problems early so that they can be minimized or eliminated. The intent of this chapter is to acquaint the nurse with the vocabulary of the prenatal period, to explain the techniques used to assess the pregnant woman, to present comprehensive information on the assessment of the woman and fetus, and to present the nursing process as a holistic approach to prenatal care.

Learning Objectives

After studying the material in this chapter, the student will be able to:

- Discuss the various methods used to diagnose pregnancy.
- Explain why early detection of pregnancy is important.
- Differentiate the presumptive, probable, and positive signs of pregnancy.
- Describe the events of the first prenatal visit.
- Explain the importance of the health history in nursing assessment.
- Describe the physical examination, and identify some normal changes of pregnancy.
- Identify the basic laboratory studies performed for early pregnancy assessment and their significance.
- List three symptoms of substance abuse in pregnant women.
- Identify three symptoms of battering in women.
- Describe subsequent assessments of the pregnant woman.

UNIT III: ADAPTATION IN THE PRENATAL PERIOD

Application of Key Terms

Match the definition in column two with the key terms in column one.

____ 1. Gestation
____ 2. Gestational age
____ 3. Gravida
____ 4. GTPALM
____ 5. Lightening
____ 6. Multigravida
____ 7. Multipara
____ 8. Nulligravida
____ 9. Nullipara
____ 10. Parity
____ 11. Primigravida
____ 12. Primipara

A. Descent of the uterus into the pelvis occurring 2 to 3 weeks before labor in primigravidas.
B. Woman who has completed two or more pregnancies to the stage of viability.
C. Woman who has delivered one fetus who reached the stage of viability.
D. Time from conception to birth, approximately 280 days.
E. Number of pregnancies reaching viability.
F. Woman who is or has been pregnant, regardless of pregnancy outcome.
G. Woman who is not now and never has been pregnant.
H. stimated age of the fetus calculated in weeks from the first day of the last menstrual period.
I. Woman who is pregnant and has been pregnant before.
J. Woman who has never carried a pregnancy to the stage of viability.
K. Woman pregnant for the first time.
L. The mnemonic system used to record the pregnancy history.

Short Answer Exercise of Critical Content

1. Place the following signs/symptoms of pregnancy in the appropriate column.

abdominal enlargement
amenorrhea
ballottement
Braxton Hicks contractions
breast tenderness
Chadwick's sign

colostrum
fatigue
fetal heartbeat
fetal movement felt by examiner
Hegar's sign

quickening
ultrasound of fetus
urinary frequency
uterine changes
Morning sickness

Presumptive Signs	Probable Signs	Positive Signs

NURSING ASSESSMENT OF THE PREGNANT WOMAN

Mrs. Simmons, a white 37 year old woman, presented to your office for her first prenatal visit. Mrs. Simmons states her last menstrual period began January 15, and a positive pregnancy test confirms she is pregnant for the sixth time. Previous pregnancy history reveals that Mrs. Simmons has had 3 spontaneous abortions because of an incompetent cervix. Her last two pregnancies were carried to term but Mrs. Simmons had to stay in bed for 3 months. She also developed gestational diabetes during her last pregnancy. Mrs. Simmons is 5ft 2in tall, weighs 190 lbs, and smokes 1 1/2 packs per day.

2. Use Nagele's rule to calculate to expected date of confinement (EDC).

3. What is Mrs. Simmons' GTPALM?

4. List four factors that places Mrs. Simmons at risk.

    a.

    b.

    c.

    d.

5. Because this is a first visit for Mrs. Simmons, list five assessments that will be conducted during this visit.

    a.

    b.

    c.

    d.

    e.

UNIT III: ADAPTATION IN THE PRENATAL PERIOD

6. Marylou is pregnant for the first time. After several visits she realized that her blood pressure, weight, and urine were measured or tested during each appointment. She ask the nurse why it is important to do these tests every time. What is the nurse's explanation for doing a blood pressure, weight, and urine dipstick at each visit?

   BP

   Wt.

   Urine

7. This was a planned pregnancy for Marylou and she is very excited. Marylou wants to know all that will happen throughout the pregnancy. Today she is asking about uterine growth, feeling the baby move and hearing the fetal heart tones for the first time. Describe where the fundus is located, fundal height, and what additional assessment can usually be made at each gestational age listed below

   a. 12 weeks gestation

   b. 16 weeks gestation

   c. 20 weeks gestation

8. Marylou questions how positive assessment data confirms the EDC. Indicate what your answer might be.

9. As Marylou progresses through her pregnancy Leopold Maneuvers are conducted. List the steps in order of performance and briefly describe each step.

10. Marylou asks what the routine schedule will be for subsequent prenatal visits. Your response would be:

NURSING ASSESSMENT OF THE PREGNANT WOMAN

Multiple Choice Exercise of Critical Content

Circle the most correct answer

1. Jana purchased an over the counter pregnancy test. The results were positive. The hormone responsible for a positive pregnancy test is:
   a. Estrogen
   b. Testosterone
   c. Lactogen
   d. Chorionic gonadotropin

2. During Jana's initial prenatal visit to confirm her pregnancy. Which of the following will be done:
   a. Urinalysis, pelvic examination, complete blood count, weight, blood pressure.
   b. Urinalysis, serology, psychiatric history, weight
   c. Pelvic examination, nutritional history, Rh determination
   d. Blood pressure, urinalysis, chest x-ray, weight, complete blood count

3. Which of the following are signs and symptoms of pregnancy Jana may notice in the first trimester?
   a. Amenorrhea, breast tenderness, easy fatigability, Goodell's sign
   b. Amenorrhea, morning sickness, enlargement and pressure of the uterus
   c. Morning sickness, breast tenderness, frequent urination, amenorrhea
   d. Breast tenderness, Goodell's sign, Chadwick's sign, amenorrhea

4. The midwife is going to do a pelvic examination on Jana. The nurse can be of most assistance to the patient by which of the following:
   a. Explaining the procedure to the patient, getting all the equipment ready, assisting the midwife
   b. Explaining the procedure to the patient, helping her find the most comfortable position, standing close to her and giving support
   c. Standing out of Jana's sight to decrease any embarrassment Jana might experience
   d. Explaining the procedure, talking to Jana during the exam to relieve Jana's anxiety

5. During the pelvic exam the nurse may suggest Jana do which of the following to decrease discomfort?
   a. Close her mouth, hold her breath when there is discomfort
   b. Open her mouth, breath quickly and pant when there is discomfort
   c. Close her mouth and breath through her nose
   d. Breathe slowly in through her nose and out through her mouth

UNIT III: ADAPTATION IN THE PRENATAL PERIOD

6. Jana has a hemoglobin of 13 gm/dL and a hematocrit of 41%. Which of the following statements about these values is most accurate?

   a. Both are within normal limits
   b. Hemoglobin is normal; hematocrit indicates physiologic anemia
   c. Hemoglobin indicates an iron deficiency anemia; hematocrit is normal
   d. Hemoglobin and hematocrit are elevated and indicate polycythemia

True and False Exercise to Critical Content

The following statements require you to assess whether or not it is true or false. If the statement is false, rewrite it so that it is correct.

1. Pregnancy cannot be diagnosed on the basis of the presumptive signs; it can only be assumed until more concrete data are available. (True/False).

2. The 9 months of pregnancy are grouped into three periods of approximately 13 weeks each; weeks 1 to 13, 14 to 28; and 29 through 42. (True/False).

3. Pelvimetry is the measurement of the dimensions and proportions of the bony pelvis to assess whether it is large enough to accommodate the delivery of an infant. (True/False).

4. An Hgb reading below 12.0g/11mL or an Hct below 35% indicates anemia in the pregnant woman. (True/False).

5. Serology tests are used to screen and diagnoses women for *Treponema pallidum* because it will cross the placenta and infect the fetus. (True/False).

6. If a pregnant woman contacts Rubella during the first 12 weeks of pregnancy the fetus could be blind, deaf, mentally retarded, or have cardiac defects. (True/False).

7. The financial, social, and psychological stress of an additional family member may precipitate or escalate acts of violence against the pregnant woman. (True/False).

NURSING ASSESSMENT OF THE PREGNANT WOMAN

8. Highrisk categories include women with previous pregnancy complications, adolescents, women older than age 35, women who are physically and emotionally abused, and women who are substance abusers. (True/False).

9. Complications often thought to be associated with cocaine use in pregnancy include preterm labor or birth, premature rupture of membranes, and sexually transmitted diseases. (True/False).

10. A prenatal assessment taken by a nurse provides no value to health maintenance during pregnancy. (True/False).

Critical Thinking Exercise

1. Eleanor Bond, age 20, is in her second pregnancy. She is African-American and lives in a government housing project. When she comes for her appointment you notice that she is overweight and is hypertensive. You are the health care worker for her and are responsible for health teaching to expectant mothers. Analyze the factors you want to investigate since she is overweight. Plan a program to help eleanor understand how and why she must reduce her caloric and salt intake. Explain why diet restriction is very important in Eleanor's situation.

2. Early in pregnancy, the expectant mother is given advice on various physical aspects of care that will enhance her well-being. Defend the advice that you will give mothers on each of the following topics: (a) care of the teeth; (b) clothes; (c) exercise; (d) relaxation-rest periods; (e) care of the breasts; and (f) bowel habits.

CHAPTER 14

Assessment of Fetal Well-Being

Overview

Fetal health largely depends on maternal condition. Attention to optimal maternal health before conception is especially important for women with preexisting disorders that contribute to perinatal problems. Knowledge of the ramifications of health problems combined with early prenatal care will help ensure the well-being of the parents and the neonate.

Learning Objectives

After studying the material in this chapter, the student will be able to:

- Describe the major modalities used for assessment of fetal well-being and when they are typically used.
- Explain why estimation of gestational age is an important component of prenatal care.
- Explain what information can be gained from amniocentesis, biophysical profile, ultrasonography, Doppler velocimetry, and fetal movement and heart rate studies.
- Explain what information is gained from nonstress testing and contraction stress testing.
- Describe nursing responsibilities related to assessment of fetal well-being.

ASSESSMENT OF FETAL WELL-BEING

Application of Key Terms

Match the definitions in column two with the key terms in column one.

_____ 1. Amniotic fluid index.
_____ 2. Auscultation acceleration test
_____ 3. Biophysical profile
_____ 4. Biparietal diameter
_____ 5. Contraction stress test
_____ 6. Crown-rump length
_____ 7. Doppler velocimetry
_____ 8. Lecithin-sphingomyelin ration
_____ 9. McDonald's measurement
_____ 10. Nonstress test
_____ 11. Percutaneous umbilical blood sampling
_____ 12. Reactivity
_____ 13. Ultrasonography
_____ 14. Vibroacoustic stimulation

A. A ratio of 2:1 is used as an indicator of fetal lung maturity.
B. Largest transverse diameter of the fetal head.
C. Use of sound waves to produce an outline of the shape of the fetus.
D. Evaluation of fetal heart rate as it relates to fetal movement.
E. Listening with a fetoscope for an increase in fetal heart tones.
F. Prenatal surveillance of the fetus at risk by use of tests of fetal well-being.
G. Stimulation of the uterine muscles by use of oxytocin to assess fetal oxygen reserves before labor.
H. An estimate of fetal gestational age based on measurement from the top of the head to the buttocks.
I. The insertion of a needle through the maternal abdomen into the umbilical cord at the site of insertion into the placenta.
J. Visualization of the pockets of amniotic fluid by ultrasound.
K. The use of an artificial larynx to provide auditor stimulus to the fetus.
L. An assessment method that uses the ultrasound stethoscope and the ultrasound transclucer.
M. Measurement of the distance from the superior border of the symphysis pubis to the top of the fundus.
N. An increase in the fetal heart rate of least 15 bpm for at least 15 seconds.

Short Answer Exercise of Critical Content

1. List four clinical indications for scheduling ultrasound to determine gestational age.

    a.

    b.

    c.

    d.

78 UNIT III: ADAPTATION IN THE PRENATAL PERIOD

2. When ultrasound is done to assess gestational age the bladder us usually full; when it is done as an adjunct to amniocentesis it is empty. Explain the rationale for this difference.

3. Compare and contrast NSTs and CSTs by completing the following table.

Parameters	Nonstress Test	Contraction Stress Test
Description of test	a	k
Environment	b	l
Client position	c	m
Length of test	d	n
Intravenous use	e	o
BP evaluation	f	p
Medication used	g	q
Monitored parameters	h	r
Test interpretation	i	s
Risk/cost	j	t

4. Mrs. Bolton, 37 years old and 17 weeks pregnant, arrives at the hospital for a scheduled amniocentesis. This is the Boltons' first baby. Mr. Bolton is with his wife, and he asks you to give him a brief explanation of the procedure; he says that their physician has explained the purpose of the test. Formulate your response to Mr. Bolton.

5. Mr. Bolton wants to know what conditions can be determined by amniocentesis.

ASSESSMENT OF FETAL WELL-BEING

6. What is the most probable reason the physician is doing an amniocentesis and why?

7. Mrs. Bolton wants to know why the physician waited until the 17th week to do the amniocentesis. Explain why.

Multiple Choice Exercise of Critical Content

Circle the most correct answer.

1. A test is scheduled to determine the lecithin/sphingomyelin (L/S) ration of the amniotic fluid. This ratio is important in assessing fetal maturity of the:
    a. Neurological system.
    b. Digestive system.
    c. Hematological system.
    d. Pulmonary system.

2. Delivery could be performed when the L/S ration is at least:
    a. 2:1.1.
    b. 1:1.8.
    c. 1:2.
    d. 1:1.5.

3. A NST is considered reactive if the examiner observes:
    a. Three contractions during a 30 minute observational period with decelerated FHT.
    b. Acceleration in the FHT of at least 15 bpm and lasting about 15 seconds with fetal movement.
    c. Acceleration in the FHT of at least 30 bpm with each contraction that lasts for 60 seconds.
    d. Decelerated FHT of at least 15 bpm and lasting about 15 to 20 seconds with each fetal movement.

4. A CST would most likely be preformed on a woman who has:
    a. A fetal L/S ration of 1.5:1 today.
    b. Just had an amniocentesis for genetic assessment.
    c. A reactive NST last week.
    d. A nonreactive NST this morning.

5. The results of a CST would be of value if there are:
   a. Continuous contractions during a 10 minute period.
   b. Three to four contractions in 30 minutes for a 60 minute period.
   c. Three to four contractions in 5 minutes for a 30 minute period.
   d. Three to four contractions in 10 minutes for a 30 minute period.

6. The CST test was negative. The nurse knows that indicates what?
   a. The frequency of the contractions were less than 3 in 10 minutes, and it was impossible to tell if late decelerations occurred.
   b. There were consistent but definite late decelerations; however they did not persist with increased amounts of oxytocin.
   c. Persistent and consistent late decelerations were occurring repeatedly with each contraction seen.
   d. There were 3 contractions observed in a 10 minute period, and no late decelerations were occurring.

7. One of the simplest noninvasive methods of monitoring fetal well-being is by using:
   a. Percutaneous umbilical blood sampling.
   b. Amniocentesis.
   c. McDonald's measurement.
   d. Contraction stress test.

8. A confirmation of gestational age is fetal movement or quickening. Primigravidas usually experience quickening between:
   a. 12 and 16 weeks.
   b. 18 and 20 weeks.
   c. 20 and 22 weeks.
   d. 10 and 12 weeks.

Matching Exercise of Critical Content

Match the diagnostic procedure with the trimester in which the procedure will most likely be performed. Some answers may be used more than once.

_____ 1. First trimester   A. Ultrasound
_____ 2. Second trimester   B. FHT
_____ 3. Third trimester   C. McDonald's measurement
                             D. Amniocentesis
                             E. NST
                             F. CST

ASSESSMENT OF FETAL WELL-BEING

Critical Thinking Exercise

1. Formulate a teaching plan for a patient who has been advised to monitor fetal activity. Incorporate the times monitoring is to take place and instruct her how to count movements. Plan guidelines you can give her in regard to a reassuring number of movements.

2. Barbara has been sent from the physician's office to have a CST test performed because of a nonreactive NST. She is very frightened and is having difficulties answering questions. Evaluate her fear and generate a plan to help her relax. Explain the procedure and the rationale for doing the CST.

3. Kathy is scheduled for a biparietal diameter of the fetal head to be measured by ultrasound. Explain at least four maternal conditions in which this test might be indicated.

CHAPTER 15

Nursing Care of the Expectant Family

Overview

Early and thorough prenatal care focuses on education aimed at maintaining well-being. The nurse is likely to have more contact with patients and their families than any other health care provider and thus must provide needed teaching. The processes of promoting health maintenance, addressing physical and psychosocial adaptations, providing support for self-care, and helping the woman maintain a healthy life-style during pregnancy are important nursing actions. This chapter focuses on nursing care in the prenatal period, with an emphasis on education.

Learning Objectives

After studying the material in this chapter, the student will be able to:

- Discuss the importance of individualizing teaching and counseling for each woman or family.

- Explain the rational for anticipatory guidance, and give an example of how it is used in caring for the expectant family.

- Discuss the importance of making referrals when indicated, and identify situations that require referrals.

- Identify causes, assessment data, interventions, and expected outcomes for the common discomforts of pregnancy.

- Identify symptoms that pregnant women must be taught to report.

- Identify risks related to employment, travel, sports, and exercise during pregnancy.

- Identify the benefits of sports and exercise during pregnancy.

- Teach pregnant women to prepare for breastfeeding.

NURSING CARE OF THE EXPECTANT FAMILY

Application of Key Terms

Match the definitions in column two with the key terms in column one.

_____ 1. Anticipatory guidance
_____ 2. Hemorrhoids
_____ 3. Homan's sign
_____ 4. Pelvic tilt
_____ 5. Kegel exercises
_____ 6. Dorsiflexion
_____ 7. Lordosis
_____ 8. Toxoplasmosis
_____ 9. Exercise-talk test

A. An infection caused by the protozoa *Toxoplasma gondii*.
B. Abnormal anterior convexity of the spine.
C. Pain in the calf on dorsiflexion of the foot.
D. Conscious tightening and relaxing of the pubococcygeal muscles.
E. The dilatation of rectal veins beneath the skin of the anal canal.
F. Pointing the toes toward the head.
G. Prepare for expected changes.
H. Exercise and talking simultaneously is a safe exercise for pregnant woman.
I. An exercise that rocks the pelvis.

Short Answer Exercise of Critical Content

1. List three possible concerns an expectant couple may have in regard to pregnancy and provide rationale(s) for each concern.

   a.

   b.

   c.

2. Anticipatory guidance is most effective when it is aimed at the learner's _____.

3. When providing anticipatory guidance, the nurse must take into account the woman's _____.

UNIT III: ADAPTATION IN THE PRENATAL PERIOD

4. Describe three exercises you would include in your teaching plan for a healthy pregnant woman.

   a.

   b.

   c.

5. Fill in the table on the discomforts of pregnancy.

Minor Discomforts	Description/Cause	Prevention/Nursing Care
Frequent Urination	a	b
Nausea	c	d
Heartburn	e	f
Fatigue	g	h
Backache	i	j
Headaches	k	l
Varicose Veins	m	n
Leg Cramps	o	p
Edema	q	r
Vaginal Discharge	s	t

NURSING CARE OF THE EXPECTANT FAMILY

6. Instruct a client about 5 of the 9 danger signals she must report immediately to her health care provider.

   a.

   b.

   c.

   d.

   e.

7. The nurse must be alert to subtle clues in the patient history and physical exam that may be suggestive of abuse. List five clues suggestive of abuse in the pregnant woman.

   a.

   b.

   c.

   d.

   e.

Multiple Choice Exercise of Critical Content

Circle the most correct answer.

1. Constipation during pregnancy is best treated by:
    a. Regular use of laxatives such as milk of magnesia
    b. Light exercise such as slow running
    c. Increased fiber and fluids in the diet
    d. Regular use of glycerine suppositories

2. Of the normal discomforts of pregnancy, which one listed below generally has its initial onset during the first part of pregnancy.

    a. Backache

    b. Dyspnea

    c. Fatigue

    d. Varicose Veins

3. Betsy is in her early months of pregnancy and complains about morning sickness. What recommendations might you make to help her?

    a. Nothing will alleviate it, and she must do her best to accept it.

    b. Eat a dry carbohydrate, such as a cracker, before arising.

    c. Take large quantities of fluids with each meal.

    d. Eat three large meals every day and avoid eating between meals.

4. Which symptom should Susan be instructed to report to her health care provider immediately?

    a. Ankle edema

    b. Heartburn

    c. Urinary Frequency

    d. Vaginal bleeding

5. Mary Jane was excited about being pregnant but at 12 weeks appears very depressed. As a nurse you know:

    a. Everyone is excited about having a baby

    b. Most women have ambivalent feelings about pregnant and mood swings are normal

    c. The baby will probably be deformed because of the depression

    d. She will not be a good mother because she is depressed and unable to care for a child

6. Paula reports that she smokes one pack of cigarettes a day. Paula has a greater chance of having a:

    a. Large for gestational age baby

    b. Small for gestational age baby

    c. Average for gestational age baby

    d. Greater chance of becoming post term

7. Greta questions how much beer she should consume during her pregnancy. The nurse should advise her to:

   a. Drink at least one glass of beer with every meal
   b. Drink at least one pint of beer a week
   c. Refrain from all alcohol consumption during pregnancy
   d. Switch from beer to wine during her pregnancy

8. Nicole is planning to go on vacation and seeks advice from the health care provider. She should be encouraged to:

   a. Go backwoods backpacking
   b. Never travel by air
   c. Travel during the second trimester
   d. Never be more than 30 minutes away from a hospital

9. The woman who is interested in breastfeeding should:

   a. Begin preparation after she delivers
   b. Be instructed to wash the nipple and areola with soap
   c. Apply drying and hardening agents such as tincture of benzoin
   d. Begin preparation early in pregnancy

10. Melody was instructed about signs of labor. True labor displays all of the signs except:

    a. Contractions felt primarily in the back
    b. Contractions sometimes relieved by walking
    c. Pink mucus discharged from vagina
    d. A leaking or gush of fluid from vagina

True and False Exercise of Critical Content

The following statements require you to assess whether or not they are true or false. If the statement is false, rewrite it so that it is correct.

1. Assessment of the entire family unit may be necessary to provide effective prenatal care. (True/False).

2. The nurse and the pregnant woman and her family plan and implement care based on the nurse's identified needs. (True/False).

3. Women who have had previous obstetric complications or losses will bring many anxieties to the current pregnancy. (True/False).

4. Clients should be referred to a nutritionist if they begin the pregnancy extremely far under or over their ideal weight. (True/False).

5. If a pregnant woman has injuries that suggest family violence, the nurse must interview her with her significant other present. (True/False).

Critical Thinking Exercise

1. Jolene arrives in labor and delivery with severe abdominal pain. She is 14 weeks pregnant. During your admission interview you learn she was kicked in the abdomen by her boyfriend. Decide what evaluation you need to conduct to refer Jolene for assistance. Formulate a plan to assist Jolene to obtain community resources.

2. Judy has been very active as a tennis player. She is participating in the state championship in six weeks. Judy has just found our she is two months pregnant. Explain to Judy what precautions she should take. Formulate a plan to help her pace herself so that she does not reach a compromised state.

CHAPTER 16

Complications of Pregnancy

Overview

Complications may occur at anytime during pregnancy. They may result from problems with the pregnancy, preexisting medical problems, infections, or substance use and abuse. An objective of prenatal care is to monitor specific parameters with the goal of averting or minimizing problems. This chapter discusses complications of pregnancy and the nurse's role of teaching clients, thereby increasing family members abilities to participate in maintaining their health.

Learning Objectives

After studying the material in this chapter, the student will be able to:

- Explain the standard medical and nursing care for the woman with hyperemesis gravidarum.
- Identify the major risks associated with placenta previa and nursing actions to reduce risk.
- List the symptoms of ectopic pregnancy and describe appropriate nursing actions when symptoms are identified.
- Describe anticipatory guidance about prenatal care the nurse should provide to the woman diagnosed with multiple gestation.
- Identify maternal risk factors when intrauterine fetal demise complicates pregnancy.
- Describe the consequences of maternal hemoglobinopathy in pregnancy.
- Discuss the major risks associated with thromboembolic disease in pregnancy.
- List the infections know to have teratogenic potential during pregnancy.
- Describe maternal and fetal or neonatal consequences of sexually transmitted disease during pregnancy.
- Discuss commonly abused substances and how their use in pregnancy affects maternal, fetal, and neonatal outcome.

Application of Key Terms

Match the definitions in column two with the key terms in column one.

1. Afibrinogenemia
2. Abruption
3. Disseminating intravascular coagulation (DIC)
4. Deep vein thrombosis
5. Ectopic pregnancy
6. Erythroblastosis
7. Gestational trophoblastic disease
8. Hemoglobinopathy
9. Hemolytic disease
10. Hemodynamic stability
11. Hydatidiform mole
12. Hyperemesis gravidarum
13. Hydrops fetalis
14. Intrauterine fetal demise (IUFD)
15. Narcotic abstinence syndrome
16. Placenta previa
17. Postterm pregnancy
18. Pulmonary embolism
19. Rh immunoglobulin (RhIgG)
20. Sensitization
21. Teratogenic infection

A. Abnormal condition of pregnancy where protracted vomiting, weight loss, and fluid and electrolyte imbalance occur.

B. Disease caused by or associated with forms of abnormal hemoglobin.

C. Complete or partial separation of the normal implanted placenta from the uterine wall.

D. A placenta that is implanted in the lower uterine segment.

E. Infections that have the ability to infect the infant during pregnancy: Toxoplasmosis, rubella, cytomegalovirus, and herpes.

F. Pregnancy that goes beyond the 42nd week of gestation.

G. A blood disorder that results from the absence or decrease of fibrinogen in the blood plasma, which becomes incoagulable.

H. Hemolytic anemia of the fetus and newborn occurring when the blood of the fetus is Rh positive and the blood of the mother is Rh negative.

I. Extreme edema of the fetus or newborn occurring in severe hemolytic disease.

J. A pathologic form of coagulation, diffuse throughout the body, in which certain clotting factors are consumed to the extent that generalized bleeding occurs.

K. Implantation of the ovum outside of the uterine cavity.

L. Disorder in cellular growth that results in the destruction of the embryo and abnormal growth of the outer layer of the blastocyst.

M. Anemia due to the premature destruction of red blood cells.

N. Gestational trophoblastic disease.

O. Death of the fetus that is retained in the uterus.

P. Formation of an abnormal clot in a venous vessel.

Q. Injection given within 72 hours to protect against sensitization.

R. When the neonate begins to exhibit signs and symptoms of narcotic withdrawal.

S. Having developed a susceptibility to a specific substance.

T. A blood clot that travels to and occludes vessels in the lungs.

U. Stable condition relating to the physical aspects of the blood circulation.

COMPLICATIONS OF PREGNANCY

Short Answer Exercise of Critical Content

1. Complete the sentences below by providing the missing word(s) in the blanks.

    a. The most common hemolytic disease of pregnancy results from _____.

    b. The _____ provides a method of testing to determine the presence of fetal cells in maternal circulation.

    c. In Rh negative mothers Rh immune globulin is administered at _____ weeks to protect against the effects of early transplacental hemorrhage.

2. Describe the cardinal sign of placenta previa:

3. June has been diagnosed with hyperemesis gravidarum. List three criteria used to diagnose this condition.

    a.

    b.

    c.

4. Joanne, age 34, gravida III, para 0, experienced two previous second-trimester abortions due to incompetent cervical os. Define incompetent cervical os.

5. List two approaches to treatment that may be presented to Joanne?

    a.

    b.

UNIT III: ADAPTATION IN THE PRENATAL PERIOD

6. Jonie, G2 P2, is Rh negative; her husband is Rh positive. Jonie's first child was Rh negative. She has just given birth to an Rh positive infant. Jonie's indirect Coombs' test is positive and so is her infants. Indicate the significance of these findings, what should be done, and why.

7. Iron deficiency anemia is diagnosed when the hemoglobin level is less than _____.

8. The most common renal problem in pregnancy is urinary tract infection. Describe how anatomical and hormonal changes in pregnancy increase the risk of urinary tract infections.

9. Cindy Smith was chemically addicted during her pregnancy. Her baby boy is exhibiting signs and symptoms of narcotic withdrawal. List the signs and symptoms baby boy Smith is displaying.

   a.

   b.

   c.

   d.

10. Josie was involved in a serious motor vehicle accident. She is 26 weeks pregnancy and has been sent to labor and delivery for observation. She has sustained multiple fractures that are now cast. You observe her closely for what condition?

COMPLICATIONS OF PREGNANCY

Multiple Choice Exercise of Critical Content

Circle the most correct answer.

1. Mrs. Carter was admitted to the hospital at 20 weeks gestation with nausea and vomiting. You would anticipate the obstetrician's treatment of choice to be:
    a. Order frequent high caloric snacks and meals.
    b. Order antiemetic, IV fluids and keep client NPO.
    c. Stimulate the patient with frequent visitors, telephone calls, and T.V. programs.
    d. Tell the patient she should not worry and continue with her routine activities.

2. Mrs. Carter responds to therapy and states she is hungry. You anticipate the obstetrician will:
    a. Continue I.V. therapy and NPO status.
    b. Order a regular diet and discontinue I.V. fluids.
    c. Begin small dry feedings prior to discontinuing fluids.
    d. Force fluids and increase the I.V. rate.

3. Mrs. Carter progresses well. Wednesday night she turns on her call light and complains of epigastric pain. You assess her for what?
    a. Intolerance of diet.
    b. Emotional distress.
    c. Inability to void.
    d. Impending labor.

4. Mrs. Carter gets up to go to the bathroom and experiences a sudden gush of bright red bleeding from the vagina. She has no other symptoms. You should:
    a. Stay with the client, auscultate FHT, and have someone call the physician.
    b. Tell the client she should rest in bed with her feet up.
    c. Try to get an order for her to use some tampons.
    d. Offer the client a glass of warm milk to drink and pain medication.

5. Mrs. Carter is diagnosed with placenta previa and fetal demise. She asks why this happened. Your best response would be:
    a. You probably strained yourself when you got up to go to the bathroom.
    b. Sometimes these things just happen.
    c. You were not ready to deliver, however the cervix dilated anyway.
    d. The placenta implanted across the cervix and for some reason the cervix dilated causing the bleeding.

6. Mrs. Carter is delivered by cesarean birth and develops disseminated intravascular coagulation (DIC). You prepare Mrs. Carter for:

    a. Routine postpartum observations and transfer to the floor.

    b. Transfer to the intensive care unit for close observation.

    c. Discharge home after 24 hours observation

    d. Transfer to surgery for complete hysterectomy.

7. The nurse anticipates the treatment of choice for DIC would be:

    a. To give hourly injections for pain.

    b. Administer cryoprecipitate as ordered.

    c. Administer heparin as ordered.

    d. Administer meds to increase cardiac output.

8. Amy is being induced because she is 43 weeks gestation. The nurse would anticipate that Amy may have:

    a. Polyhydramnios, small baby and a short labor with rapid delivery.

    b. Small baby that is not premature and a long hard delivery.

    c. Oligohydramnios; meconium-stained fluid, macrosomia, and placental insufficiency.

    d. Polyhydramnios, clear fluid, microsomia, and shoulder dystocia.

9. Betty serves food on a cafeteria line. One day she complains of a very sore leg and she cannot walk. Because she is 24 weeks pregnant she goes to see her midwife. Betty most likely will be diagnosed with:

    a. Hydramnios.

    b. Deep vein thrombosis.

    c. Placenta previa.

    d. Pulmonary embolism.

10. June was exposed to rubella during her first trimester. Her baby is at risk for what possible defect?

    a. Cerebral calcification.

    b. Encephalitis.

    c. Sepsis.

    d. Deafness.

COMPLICATIONS OF PREGNANCY

Matching Exercise of Critical Content

One of the purposes of prenatal care is to monitor the physiological changes of pregnancy to detect any problems. Many of the complications that occur have similar signs and symptoms. However, some signs and symptoms are specific to probable pathologic states. Match a complication of pregnancy you would be concerned about if you knew the patient was experiencing the signs or symptom.

	Signs and Symptoms	Complication
_____	1. Hematocrit less than 30 in a Greek patient.	A. Preterm labor
_____	2. Persistent urinary track infection in an African American patient.	B. Thalassemia
		C. Ectopic pregnancy
_____	3. History of second trimester painless spontaneous abortion.	D. Severe preeclampsia
_____	4. Shoulder pain associated with spotting.	E. Sickle cell trait
_____	5. Large for gestational age without fetal heart tone.	F. Incompetent cervix
		G. Placenta previa
_____	6. Second trimester painless vaginal bleeding.	H. Hydatidiform mole
_____	7. Large for dates uterine size after twenty weeks.	I. Multiple gestation
_____	8. Cervical change before 37 weeks.	
_____	9. Nausea and vomiting with epigastric pain in the second half of pregnancy.	

True and False Exercise of Critical Content

The following statements require you to assess whether or not they are true or false. If the statement is false, rewrite it so that it is correct.

1. Gestational complications present a range of maternal, fetal, and neonatal consequences. Examples of gestational complications include; hyperemesis gravidarus, spontaneous abortion, IUFD, and incompetent cervix. (True/False).

2. In most cases, complications in pregnancy require mobilization of appropriate medical and nursing care. (True/False).

3. A decreased immunologic response to infection is one of the normal physiologic adaptations to pregnancy. (True/False).

4. Maternal infections should be readily treated with antibiotics. (True/False).

5. Part of the nursing responsibility may be to teach the pregnant woman how to prevent infections; what the outcomes of infections may be to the woman, her fetus, and her neonate; and how to care for herself if the condition is chronic. (True/False).

6. Chemical addiction and illegal drug use causes significant problems in the perinatal period. (True/False).

7. All pregnant women should be screened for chemical use, including nonprescription drugs, coffee, cigarettes, and alcohol. (True/False).

8. If a mother has been identified as a drug addict, neonatal personnel should be notified in advance of the birth so that preparations may be made for a high-risk neonate. (True/False).

9. The most frequent cause of trauma in pregnant women is motor vehicle accidents, although other trauma includes domestic violence, falls, and burns. (True/False).

10. Trauma to a pregnant women usually is an indication for immediate termination of the pregnancy. (True/False).

Critical Thinking Exercise

1. When a patient is admitted for preterm labor monitoring she is usually experiencing increased stress and anxiety. Because this is not the ideal situation for learning, it is helpful to give written instructions for the patient to review after she goes home. Generate a teaching tool to give to the patient who has been placed on tocolytic therapy to go home on self-monitoring.

2. Belinda, a 27-year old, gravida II, para I, experienced spotting beginning at 32 weeks gestation. Ultrasound indicated placenta previa. Structure a plan of care for Belinda. Include probable health care provider orders and procedures.

3. Sarah comes to labor and delivery at 32 weeks in labor. While taking her admission history you learn she is a crack user and has had no prenatal care. The health care provider orders blood work for HIV/AIDS which comes back positive. Evaluate your feelings about Sarah's situation. Decide upon a plan to refer Sarah to appropriate resources. Structure a communication method to alert staff of the necessary precautions to take when caring for Sarah and her baby.

CHAPTER 17

Nutrition During Pregnancy

Overview

An important determinant of the woman's well-being and that of her fetus is her nutritional status. Counseling and nutrition education are necessary to ensure normal fetal growth and development. Nurses must appreciate the importance of nutrition and be knowledgeable about how the normal physiologic changes during pregnancy relate to nutritional needs. This chapter presents basic information on the effects of maternal nutritional status on the course and outcome of pregnancy and describes daily nutritional requirements during pregnancy.

Learning Objectives

After studying the material in this chapter, the student will be able to:

- Identify steps to assess, maintain, and promote the nutritional status of pregnant women.

- Identify and relate nutritional risk factors during pregnancy.

- Use dietary guidelines in helping pregnant women meet their nutritional needs.

- Specify recommended daily intake of vitamins and minerals that are particularly important during pregnancy.

- Offer appropriate nutrition counseling to pregnant women based on assessment of economic, religious, and cultural factors.

Application of Key Terms

Match the definitions in column two with the key terms in column one.

_____ 1. Body mass index
_____ 2. Calorie
_____ 3. Folic acid
_____ 4. Iron cost
_____ 5. Iron deficiency anemia
_____ 6. Kilocalorie
_____ 7. Megadose
_____ 8. Nutritional requirement
_____ 9. Pica (geophagia)
_____ 10. Recommended Dietary Allowances (RDA)

A. Craving during pregnancy to eat substances that are not food, such as chalk, clay, starch, glue, toothpaste.

B. Unit of measure for heat; a large calorie.

C. Standards by age and sex group for intake of major nutrients; serve as guidelines for maintaining health through nutrition.

D. Unit of heat.

E. Member of the vitamin B complex.

F. Amount of a substance (vitamin) that is at least 10 times greater than the RDA.

G. Foods necessary for good health, including a variety and amount necessary to maintain ideal weight.

H. Approximately 3 mg absorbed iron is required daily during pregnancy.

I. A common nutritional disorder of pregnancy that imposes a limit on the body's ability to transport oxygen to the tissue.

J. Ratio of weight to height.

Short Answer Exercise of Critical Content

1. List five potential risk factors affecting nutritional status during pregnancy.

    a.

    b.

    c.

    d.

    e.

NUTRITION DURING PREGNANCY

2. Fill in the blanks in the following paragraph that describes the medical condition of anemia.

   Mild or moderate anemia in the nonpregnant female is defined as having a hemoglobin level _____ g/dL or a hematocrit level _____ vol %. Severe anemia is either a nonpregnant or pregnant female is defined as having a hemoglobin level _____ g/dL or a hematocrit _____ vol %. In the pregnant female, mild or moderate anemia is defined as having a hemoglobin level _____ g/dL or a hematocrit of _____ vol%.

3. Describe the information obtained when performing an assessment of nutritional status for a pregnant client.

4. Decide what your response would be to a woman who asks why alcohol use and caffeine intake should be avoided during pregnancy.

Multiple Choice Exercise of Critical Content

Circle the most correct answer.

1. Darnell is placed on iron tablets. When supplementary iron is given, the patient should be told to expect.
   a. Diarrhea
   b. Black stools with blood streaks
   c. Black stools and possible constipation
   d. Heartburn

2. Heartburn during pregnancy results from:
   a. Increased work load of the heart
   b. Increased stomach acidity
   c. Increased peristalsis
   d. Decreased gastric motility with reflux

3. During the second and third trimesters of pregnancy, Betty Joe will need how many additional calories over her nonpregnant needs?
   a. 500 kcal/d
   b. 300 kcal/d
   c. 900 kcal/d
   d. 1000 kcal/d

4. The two most important substances Betty Joe should increase in her diet are:
   a. Vitamins and sodium
   b. Calcium and sodium
   c. Protein and iron
   d. Vitamins and minerals

5. Daktara is a vegetarian. What nutrients may be lacking in a vegetarian diet?
   a. Protein and calcium
   b. Iron and folic acid
   c. Minerals and calories
   d. Carbohydrates and Iron

6. Low-income pregnant women are especially vulnerable to nutritional deficiency and should be referred to the:
   a. SPCA program
   b. HOPE program
   c. ABC program
   d. WIC program

NUTRITION DURING PREGNANCY

Matching Exercise of Critical Content

Match the following nutrient with the appropriate RDA required during pregnancy.

	Nutrient		RDA
_____	1. Vitamin A	A.	80 mg
_____	2. Vitamin D	B.	4 mcg
_____	3. Vitamin E	C.	1000 mcg RE
_____	4. Vitamin C	D.	15 mcg
_____	5. Folacin	E.	Additional 400 mg
_____	6. Vitamin B12	F.	175 mg
_____	7. Calcium	G.	20 mg
_____	8. Zinc	H.	800 mcg
_____	9. Iodine	I.	10 mg TE

True and False Exercise of Critical Content

The following statements require you to assess whether or not they are true or false. If the statement is false, rewrite it so that it is correct.

1. All health professionals involved in the delivery of prenatal nutrition services should be able to counsel on nutrient needs and recommended diet during pregnancy and infancy. (True/False).

2. Some maternal physiologic adjustments have effects on overall metabolism and are the basis for the decreased nutritional requirements. (True/False).

3. Even a woman whose nutritional status is excellent will complete a pregnancy with a deficit in available iron if her dietary intake is not supplemented. (True/False).

4. Vitamins and mineral supplementation is recommended to all pregnant women. (True/False).

5. The health history is especially important in identifying factors that put pregnant women at nutritional risk. (True/False).

6. Appropriate weight gain during pregnancy is essential to the continued good health of the mother and normal development of the fetus. (True/False).

7. Individual patients known to be at high nutritional risk, such as adolescents, impoverished women, or those with previously identified nutritional problems, will require additional time for individualized teaching and counseling. (True/False).

8. The woman's cultural background, socioeconomic status, and developmental level directly influence her dietary patterns and her overall nutritional status. (True/False).

Critical Thinking Exercise

1. Formulate a nutritionally adequate diet for a pregnant woman using commonly available foods. In your diet plan explain the specific changes that might need to be made for each of these clients: teenager, African-American, Asian-American, and Hispanic.

2. Contact the local health department and attend a WIC counseling session. Analyze the criteria that must be met in order to qualify for the program. Generate a list of foods/commodities available on this program.

3. Structure a teaching plan for Lisa age 18, focusing on calorie intake and recommended weight gain pattern for the three trimesters of pregnancy. Lisa is 5 feet tall and her prepregnancy weight was 175 pounds.

UNIT IV: ADAPTATION IN THE INTRAPARTUM PERIOD

CHAPTER 18

Comprehensive Education for Childbirth

Overview

An understanding of the content of current childbirth education programs enables the nurse to support families who are prepared. Knowledge of specific techniques and approaches for coping with labor provides the nurse with the ability to support the unprepared woman and her family. This chapter provides information about the content and changing nature of comprehensive childbirth education.

Learning Objectives

After studying the material in this chapter, the student will be able to:

- Describe the major trends and influences in childbirth education.
- Recognize ways in which the childbirth education movement has affected obstetric nursing care.
- Identify the documented benefits of childbirth education.
- List the organizations involved in childbirth education and certification of childbirth educators.
- Outline the basic components of childbirth education programs.
- Describe commonly used labor-coping techniques, and explain the underlying theory of their effectiveness.
- Explain the key points of appropriate nursing care of women using specific labor-coping techniques.
- Explain how the nurse can serve as an advocate for parents wishing to follow a birth plan.
- Discuss examples of programs designed for groups with particular needs for education during the childbearing year.
- Discuss nursing roles in childbirth education.

UNIT IV: ADAPTATION IN THE INTRAPARTUM PERIOD

Application of Key Terms

Match the definition in column two with the key terms in column one.

_____ 1. Birth plan
_____ 2. Conditioned response
_____ 3. Effleurage
_____ 4. Hyperventilation
_____ 5. Preconception education
_____ 6. Progressive relaxation
_____ 7. Psychoprophylaxis
_____ 8. Sensate focus
_____ 9. Signal or cleansing breath
_____ 10. Visualization

A. Light, rhythmic stroking of the abdomen during labor.
B. Increased, forced respiration that may induce dizziness or fainting.
C. Response acquired as a result of training and repetition.
D. An expression of consumers preferences for care during labor and early postpartum.
E. A method taught to enable the achievement of a relaxed state.
F. A technique of consciously using calming and peaceful mental and visual images to maintain emotional equilibrium.
G. Focused concentration on a particular sensory stimulus to alter and diminish pain perception.
H. A deep inhalation through the nose and exhalation through the mouth.
I. Education prior to pregnancy.
J. Mind prevention to eliminate or reduce perception of pain.

Short Answer Exercise of Critical Content

1. Identify three components of prenatal education programs.

    a.

    b.

    c.

2. List the three main goals of childbirth education.

    a.

    b.

    c.

3. You are preparing for a childbirth education class where you will teach parents relaxation techniques. In simple terms, develop a portion of a teaching plan which indicates the differences between the following techniques:

(a) Imagery or visualization   versus   (b) Sensate focus

(c) Progressive relaxation   versus   (d) Neuromuscular dissociation

(e) Gentle massage   versus   (f) Effleurage

Multiple Choice Exercise of Critical Content

Circle the most correct answer.

1. Childbirth classes prepare a woman to expect that she:
   a. Will not be able to handle labor contractions if she does the breathing techniques
   b. Will be coached by the physician and the nursing staff during labor.
   c. Will receive medications and usually a general anesthesia.
   d. Will experience an unusually satisfying feeling of accomplishment when her baby is born.

2. The purpose of teaching exercise for childbirth is:
   a. To develop strong abdominal muscles.
   b. To teach tension and holding back techniques.
   c. To promote good posture.
   d. To teach various breathing and relaxation techniques.

3. Mary Jane has been in labor for 15 hours. Slow progress is being made and she is uncomfortable and frustrated. Her husband is supportive but seems unsure of what to do. What measure would you not suggest to this couple?
   a. Offer ice chips.
   b. Reposition with pillows.
   c. Offer a chocolate milkshake.
   d. Reposition with pillows.

4. You teach Mary Jane to lightly stroke her abdomen during a contraction. This method is known as:

   a. Hyperventilation.

   b. Effleurage.

   c. Sensate focus.

   d. Psychoprophylaxis.

5. Sineta has come to labor and delivery in early labor. She has not attended any childbirth classes. What simple technique can the nurse easily teach her to help Sineta through the early stages of labor?

   a. Birth plan.

   b. Hyperventilation.

   c. Slow chest breathing.

   d. Conditioned response.

Matching Exercise of Critical Content

Match the contribution to childbirth education with the person or association.

_____ 1. Author of Childbirth Without Fear.

_____ 2. Obstetrician who promoted psychoprophylactic method.

_____ 3. Promoted husband coached childbirth and deep relaxation techniques.

_____ 4. Promotes parent education programs as one of its services.

_____ 5. Developed teacher training and certification for childbirth educators.

_____ 6. Developed guidelines for scope of childbirth education and competencies of educators.

A. Dr. Ferdinand Lamaze

B. Dr. Robert Bradley

C. Dr. Grantly Dick-Read

D. International Childbirth Educators Association

E. American Red Cross

F. Association of Women's Health Obstetric, and Neonatal Nurses.

True and False Exercise of Critical Content

The following statements require you to assess whether or not they are true or false. If the statement is false, rewrite it so that it is correct.

1. Childbirth practices have been influenced by trends in medical care and more recently by a trend toward more consumer choice about how birth is managed. (True/False).

2. Educating the woman and her family about childbirth and helping the woman plan for childbirth and communicate her concerns and desires to the health care team has no implications for nursing. (True/False).

3. Research to date has focused on measuring outcomes that are strongly affected by factors outside the influence of childbirth education techniques. (True/False).

4. The goals of childbirth education focus on providing information and techniques useful to the woman and her support person as she copes with labor and birth. (True/False).

5. Preparation for childbirth includes health education, which ideally should start in the preconception period, address groups with specialized learning needs, family members, and education for the transition to parenthood. (True/False).

Critical Thinking Exercise

1. Elise and Joe ask you why they should take childbirth preparation classes. Explain to them four key components included in most classes and why the classes would be helpful to them. Apprise Elise and Joe of things they should look for when selecting a class.

2. Compare/contrast the different methods of childbirth education classes that are available to the general public.

3. Laura obtains prenatal care in her 8th month of pregnancy. Formulate a plan to provide her with a crash course in childbirth education.

CHAPTER 19

The Process of Labor And Birth
Maternal and Fetal Adaptations

Overview

The process of labor and birth is a fairly predictable sequence of events that usually occurs in a harmonious fashion and results in a healthy mother and neonate. Nursing care during childbirth can change dramatically in minutes as the woman moves through the stages of labor. Nurses must have a thorough understanding of the anatomic and physiologic changes that occur during labor and birth to allow for the provision of appropriate and effective care. This chapter reviews the anatomic and physiologic changes of labor and birth and discusses behavioral changes in the woman and the fetus.

Learning Objectives

After studying the material in this chapter, the student will be able to:

- Describe the dynamic relationship between the bony pelvis, the fetus, and the pelvic and perineal muscles and ligaments during the process of labor and birth.

- Define and describe the stages of labor.

- Describe the cardinal movements of the fetus during labor and birth.

- Explain the possible causes of onset of labor.

- Describe the process of cervical effacement and dilatation and their significance for progress in labor.

- Discuss maternal psychophysiologic responses during labor and birth.

- List signs of labor and distinguish between false and true labor.

- Outline maternal physiologic and behavioral adaptations during labor and birth.

- Outline fetal physiologic and behavioral adaptations during labor and birth.

THE PROCESS OF LABOR AND BIRTH

Application of Key Terms

Match the definitions in column two with the key terms in column one.

_____ 1. Bregma
_____ 2. Cephalic
_____ 3. Cephalopelvic disproportion
_____ 4. Contraction
_____ 5. Crowning
_____ 6. Dilatation
_____ 7. Dilatation and curettage
_____ 8. Effacement
_____ 9. Engagement
_____ 10. Fontanelle
_____ 11. Labor
_____ 12. Lie
_____ 13. Linea terminalis
_____ 14. Mentum
_____ 15. Molding
_____ 16. Occiput
_____ 17. Position
_____ 18. Presentation
_____ 19. Sinciput
_____ 20. Station
_____ 21. True pelvis
_____ 22. Vertex

A. Rhythmic contraction and relaxation of the uterine muscles with progressive effacement and dilatation of the cervix.

B. Cephalic or head.

C. Measurement of fetal descent into the bony pelvis in relation to the ischial spines.

D. Point in labor at which the widest diameter of the fetal presenting part passes through the pelvic inlet.

E. Pertaining to the head.

F. Relationship of the long axis of the fetus to the long axis of the mother.

G. Relation of the fetal presenting part to the maternal pelvis.

H. Periodic, rhythmic tightening of the uterine musculature during labor.

I. Softening, thinning, and shortening of the cervix.

J. Position of the fetus as described by the fetal part that appears first at the pelvic outlet.

K. Distention of the perineum by the largest diameter of the presenting part.

L. Unfused areas between fetal skull bones that are covered with strong connective tissue.

M. Normal process by which the fetal head is shaped during labor as it passes through the tight birth canal.

N. Opening or enlargement of the cervix.

O. Condition in which the infant's head is of a shape, size, or position that prevents it from passing through the mother's pelvis.

P. Procedure in which the uterine cervix is dilated and the endometrium of the uterus is scraped away.

Q. The lower back portion of the head.

R. Front of the head formed by the frontal bone.

S. Separates the true pelvis from the false pelvis.

T. Brow.

U. Chin

V. Lies below the linea terminalis.

UNIT IV: ADAPTATION IN THE INTRAPARTUM PERIOD

Short Answer Exercise of Critical Content

1. Four factors, commonly known as the "four Ps" are of critical importance in the process of childbirth. List the "four Ps" and give a brief explanation of their importance.

    a.

    b.

    c.

    d.

2. Complete the following information about pelvic measurements.

	Location	Measurement
Diagonal Conjugate	a.	
Obstetric Conjugate	b.	
Biischial Diameter	c.	

3. List four techniques used to determine presentation and position.

    a.

    b.

    c.

    d.

THE PROCESS OF LABOR AND BIRTH

4. The fetal skull is composed of eight bones. The four bones in the upper part of the cranium are separated by membranous interspaces called _____. The intersection of these interspaces is know as _____.

5. Complete the following information about the diameters of the fetal skull.

	Location	Measurement
Suboccipitobregmatic diameter	a.	
Biparietal diameter	b.	

6. Breech presentations are divided into three types. List each type and briefly define each.

   a.

   b.

   c.

7. Indicate the correct order of the cardinal movements of labor and birth.

   _____ a. Internal rotation
   _____ b. Descent
   _____ c. Extension
   _____ d. External rotation and expulsion
   _____ e. Flexion
   _____ f. Restitution

8. Explain the following abbreviations.

   a. LOA

   b. LOP

   c. RSA

   d. RMA

   e. LOT

   f. RSP

9. Explain the possible causes of labor according to each of the four theories listed below.

   a. The uterine stretch theory.

   b. The pressure theory of labor initiation.

   c. Hormonal Initiation Theory.

   d. Uterine Decidua Activation Theory.

10. List and briefly define the four stages of labor.

    a.

    b.

    c.

    d.

THE PROCESS OF LABOR AND BIRTH

11. Julie has just begun her 36th week of pregnancy. Inform her of certain phenomena that may alert her to approaching labor.

    a.

    b.

    c.

    d.

    e.

12. List the signs of true labor.

    a.

    b.

    c.

Multiple Choice Exercise of Critical Content

Circle the most correct answer.

Joan was admitted to the labor and delivery area of a local hospital at 0700 hours in active labor. The nurse assesses Joan and does a vaginal examination.

1. A vaginal examination was done to determine which of the following?
    a. Cervical effacement
    b. Cervical dilation
    c. Type of presentation and fetal position
    d. All of the above

2. Joan's cervix is 4 cm and 80% effaced. You know that effacement means:
   a. Elongation of the cervical canal
   b. Obliteration of the cervical canal
   c. Thickening of the cervical canal
   d. Dilatation of the cervical canal

3. Joan continues to progress in labor and after the next vaginal examination the nurse indicates that the fetal head is engaged. Engagement of the head means that:
   a. The head is crowning
   b. The head is molded
   c. The saggital suture is in the right oblique diameter
   d. The largest diameter has entered the inlet of the pelvis

4. The portion of the fetus which engages at the superior strait refers to what is called:
   a. The position of the fetus
   b. The presentation of the fetus
   c. The crowning of the fetus
   d. The station of the fetus

5. Joan's contractions are 3 minutes apart. To determine the frequency of contractions, the nurse monitors the time:
   a. From the beginning of one contraction until the beginning of the next.
   b. From the end of one contraction until the end of the next.
   c. From the beginning of one contraction until the end of that contraction.
   d. From the end of one contraction until the beginning of the next contraction.

6. When is the second stage of labor considered to be terminated?
   a. When the cervix is completely dilated.
   b. When contractions occur at 2 to 3 minutes intervals.
   c. When the baby is delivered.
   d. When the placenta is delivered.

7. Joan's baby was delivered in an ROA position. The fetal position considered most favorable for both mother and baby:
   a. Left occiput anterior.
   b. Right occiput anterior.
   c. Left occiput posterior.
   d. Right occiput transverse.

THE PROCESS OF LABOR AND BIRTH

8. The third stage of Joan's labor is the period of time from:
   a. 7 to 10 cm. dilatation.
   b. Full dilatation to the birth of the baby.
   c. Birth of the baby to birth of the placenta.
   d. Birth of the placenta to one hour postpartum.

True and False Exercise of Critical Content

The following statements require you to assess whether or not they are true or false. If the statement is false, rewrite it so that it is correct.

1. A decrease in the effectiveness of uterine contractions or an increase in the size of the fetus, may delay the process of labor. (True/False).

2. The fetus as passenger must undergo a series of unpredictable and unsynchronized maneuvers to descend through the maternal pelvis. (True/False).

3. In most cases the diameter of the shoulders is larger than the head. (True/False).

4. Nausea, vomiting, increased irritability, and even a sense of panic may occur when the woman is in the transition phase. (True/False).

5. The membranes may rupture at any time before or during the first stage of labor, but occasionally they remain intact until the cervix is completely dilated. (True/False).

6. Primigravidas usually experience about 8 hours of labor while multigravidas will experience 14 to 15 hours. (True/False).

7. Early signs of labor are often subtle, and both the woman and the nurse may be unsure of their significance. (True/False).

8. The fetus experiences drastic changes in pressure, position, and posture, which require complex physiologic adaptations. (True/False).

9. During the third stage of labor maternal physiologic stability is achieved, but the psychological adaptation to parenthood is just beginning. (True/False).

10. The psyche, or maternal adaptation, must allow the woman to cope with the pain and physical demands of labor so that she can maintain physiologic and emotional balance and can actively push the fetus out during the second stage of labor. (True/False).

Critical Thinking Exercise

1. Compare and contrast labor curves of three of the following clients: A primigravida, a multigravida, an unmedicated primigravida, a primigravida receiving intravenous analgesia, a primigravida receiving epidural anesthesia, and a client delivered by cesarean birth for failure to progress.

2. Cassie calls the health care provider's office to state she is having pain in her abdomen. She is 39 weeks pregnant and thinks she is in labor. Evaluate Cassie's situation. Decide what questions you need to ask her. Formulate a plan to help Cassie distinguish true labor from false labor.

3. You are teaching a prenatal childbirth class. Structure an outline to teach the participants the signs and symptoms of labor.

CHAPTER 20

Nursing Care in Normal Labor
First Stage

Overview

Nursing care of families during labor focuses on maintaining normal physiologic and emotional status of all family members - woman, fetus and newborn, and father or significant others - as they move through the rapid changes of the intrapartum period. The labor nurse individualizes care to meet the family's needs and desires within the health care providers framework of obstetric management. Labor and birth, as a progression of normal physiologic and psychological events, require expert nursing assessment skills and timely problem identification, intervention, and evaluation on a continuous basis. This chapter focuses on nursing care during the first stage of labor.

Learning Objectives

After studying the material in this chapter, the student will be able to:

- Discuss the application of the nursing process in caring for a woman in active labor and her family.
- Identify the signs of labor.
- Distinguish between false and true labor.
- Outline the differences between physiologic and active management of labor.
- Explain the technique of timing and palpating uterine contractions.
- Describe nonpharmacologic strategies for pain relief during labor.
- Outline the standard of nursing care for assessment of the woman in the latent, active, and transition phases of labor.
- Describe the advantages and disadvantages of electronic fetal monitoring.

Application of Key Terms

Match the definitions in column two with the key terms in column one.

_____ 1. Active management of labor
_____ 2. Active phase of labor
_____ 3. Bloody show
_____ 4. Caput (succedaneum)
_____ 5. Effleurage
_____ 6. Electronic Fetal monitoring
_____ 7. Intrapartum
_____ 8. Latent phase of labor
_____ 9. Molding
_____ 10. Prodromal labor
_____ 11. Transition phase of labor

A. The last segment of active phase of labor from 8 to 10 cm. of cervical dilatation.

B. Light, rhythmic stroking of the abdomen during labor.

C. Period from initiation of true labor contractions through 3 to 4 cm. of cervical dilatation.

D. Blood-tinged mucous discharge from the vagina that accompanies dilatation of the cervix.

E. Swelling produced on the fetal head during labor.

F. Period preceding labor when lightening occurs and increased pressure in the pelvis is felt.

G. Occurring during labor or birth.

H. Normal process by which the fetal head is shaped during labor as it passes through the birth canal.

I. An instrument that allows for intermittent or continuous monitoring of FHR and the duration and frequency of uterine contractions.

J. The stage of labor from 5 to 7 cm. of cervical dilatation distinguished by a marked change in pace and intensity of the process.

K. Interventions aimed at promoting labor.

Short Answer Exercise of Critical Content

1. Reba calls the labor unit because she believes she is in labor. She states, My pains started three hours ago and they are about 10 minutes apart. Should I come to the hospital? Reba's due date is this week. What other information would you need to ask Reba in order to advise her?

2. Based upon the information you obtain, you ask Reba to come to the hospital. What other information can you now obtain to further confirm that she is in labor?

NURSING CARE IN NORMAL LABOR

3. You perform a vaginal examination on Reba to help you assess her labor status. Follow the example of the first assessment and complete the chart with information you would need to obtain.

Status of membranes	Intact, ruptured, or bulging
Status of cervix	
Fetal presentation	
Fetal station	
Engagement	

4. Under what circumstance(s) is a vaginal examination contraindicated?

5. Reba progresses in labor. Describe how you assess the intensity of uterine contractions.

6. How would you assess the frequency of Reba's contractions?

7. Describe how you would assess the duration of Reba's contractions.

8. While caring for Reba her membranes rupture. What observations should you make and note in her chart?

   a.

   b.

   c.

   d.

   e.

UNIT IV: ADAPTATION IN THE INTRAPARTUM PERIOD

9. Place a check beside the conditions for which you would notify the health care provider.

   _____ a. Maternal pulse 90

   _____ b. Maternal B/P of 130/70

   _____ c. Maternal resp. of 28

   _____ d. FHR of 170 for over 10 min.

   _____ e. Contractions of 70 second duration for a client on oxytocin

   _____ f. Less than 30 seconds between contractions for a client on oxytocin

   _____ g. Palpable or visible fetal cord in the vagina

10. Complete the following chart regarding first stage labor. Indicate in which phase the finding would typically occur by placing an X in the appropriate column. The first one is completed for you.

Findings	Latent Phase	Active Phase	Transition
A. Cervical dilatation 3cm	X		
B. Urge to push			
C. Cervical dilatation 9cm			
D. Excited but relaxed			
E. Seriousness, sense of purpose			
F. Shaking and chills			
G. Fear of being left alone, but interacts very little			
H. Change from relaxation to tension			
I. Inability to focus, confusion			
J. Cervical dilatation 6cm			

NURSING CARE IN NORMAL LABOR

Multiple Choice Exercise of Critical Content

Circle the most correct answer.

1. Beverly is being admitted to labor and delivery. When admitting an obstetric patient in early labor to the unit, the first thing to do is to see that:

    a. The perineal shave is done immediately.

    b. Beverly's clothes are properly checked.

    c. Good rapport is established with Beverly and her significant other.

    d. Temperature, pulse, respirations, blood pressure, and FHR are taken.

2. It is important that an admission temperature, pulse, and respiration be taken during Beverly's admission because:

    a. It is a hospital routine.

    b. Baseline data needs to be identified.

    c. The patient expects it.

    d. Beverly probably has an elevated temp.

3. Beverly is unsure if her membranes have ruptured. During the initial vaginal examination, you test her with Nitrazine paper. If Beverly's membranes are ruptured, the paper will turn:

    a. Red

    b. Yellow

    c. Green

    d. Blue

4. Beverly should be encouraged to void every two hours because:

    a. A full bladder may hinder labor by preventing the presenting parts from descending.

    b. Several urine specimens are required during labor.

    c. Need to prevent the patient from being catheterized at the time of delivery.

    d. Need to test the urine for spillage of acetone or albumin.

5. As a general rule, solid foods are withheld during labor because:

    a. The emptying time of the stomach is markedly prolonged during labor.

    b. There is a danger that solid particles of food might be aspirated if the woman vomits.

    c. Normal labor is short enough so that a patient will suffer no harm if food is withheld.

    d. All of the above are correct.

6. Janice asks you if she is in labor. Her due date is tomorrow an she has been experiencing contractions all night. What can you tell her to do that might help her determine if she is in true or false labor?
    a. Rush to the Birthing Center immediately to be checked.
    b. Go to bed immediately and elevate her feet.
    c. Walk, since it often makes false labor go away.
    d. Take some pain medication and wait one hour to see what happens.

7. Before placing the patient on the electronic fetal monitor, the nurse assess the contractions by:
    a. Placing her fingertips on the woman's uterine fundus.
    b. Placing her whole hand on the uterine fundus.
    c. Pushing her finger into the mother's abdomen below the umbilicus.
    d. Placing her fingertips on the woman's lower uterine segment.

8. Following a completed admission assessment, the nurse:
    a. Continues to monitor the patient.
    b. Notifies the health care provider of findings.
    c. Sends the patient to x-ray for pelvimetry.
    d. Starts an intravenous drip of oxytocin.

9. If the woman and fetus are determined to be low risk, the FHR pattern is assessed and documented:
    a. Every 30 minutes in latent phase.
    b. Every 15 minutes during active and transition phase.
    c. Every 30 minutes during the active and transition phase.
    d. Every 10 minutes during the second stage of labor.

10. The latent phase of labor is considered prolonged if it exceeds.
    a. 10 hours for primigravidas or 8 hours for the multipara.
    b. 5 hours for primigravidas or 6 hours for the multipara.
    c. 14 hours for primigravidas or 20 hours for the multipara.
    d. 20 hours for the primigravida or 14 hours for the multipara.

Matching Exercise of Critical Content

Match the correct nursing intervention with the client situation.

	Client Situation		Nursing Intervention
_____	1. Possible slow amniotic membrane leak.	A.	Auscultate fetal heart rate.
_____	2. Auscultated decelerations in fetal heart rate.	B.	Have client blow out breaths of air through pursed lips.
_____	3. Rapid, deep breathing; dizziness; numbness of the lips.	C.	Initiate continuous external fetal monitoring.
_____	4. Artificial rupture of membranes.	D.	Have client breathe into a paper bag or cupped hands.
_____	5. Urge to push before full cervical dilatation.	E.	Apply sacral pressure.
_____	6. Back labor, increased sacral pain.	F.	Test fluid on pad or vaginal mucosa with Nitrazine paper.

True and False Exercise of Critical Content

The following statements require you to assess whether or not they are true or false. If the statement is false, rewrite it so that it is correct.

1. The period surrounding the onset of labor is often a time of acute and/or severe anxiety and crises. (True/False).

2. A woman in the latent phase of labor often expresses feelings of excitement and relief. (True/False).

3. The major goals of nursing care during the latent phase of labor are to reinforce self-care activities and review relaxation and pain control techniques. (True/False).

4. Close monitoring of physiologic and behavioral adaptations is essential as the stressors of labor are intensified. (True/False).

5. The primary goals of nursing care during the active phase of labor include the same goals as during the latent phase. (True/False).

6. The dramatic changes observed during the transition phase of labor herald the impending birth of the neonate. (True/False).

7. The primary aims of nursing care during transition include monitoring maternal and fetal physiologic status, progress of dilatation, fetal descent, and coaching the woman. (True/False).

8. The nurse needs to take-over the role of the coach during the transition period (True/False).

Critical Thinking Exercise

1. Marlene arrives in labor and delivery claiming her membranes have ruptured. Analyze the status of Marlene's statement. Generate questions you would want to ask her. Decide what test/procedures you would want to perform.

2. James, Marlene's boyfriend, has accompanied Marlene to labor and delivery. He appears somewhat ill at ease and in the way. Plan what you can do to help James during the birth process. Explain how he can assist in supporting Marlene. Structure support and comfort measures you can teach him.

CHAPTER 21

Nursing Care in Normal Birth
Second Stage of Labor Through Recovery

Overview

The physiologic and behavioral changes of the first stage of labor become increasingly dramatic in the second stage, as the process of fetal descent becomes dominant. The nurse continues assessment, interventions, and evaluations of family care. This chapter presents the nursing care for labor, delivery, and immediate post- partum care.

Learning Objectives

After studying the material in this chapter, the student will be able to:

- Discuss the application of the nursing process in caring for a woman and her family during the second stage of labor through recovery.

- Describe the types, indications, risks, and benefits of an episiotomy.

- Assess the placenta, cord, and fetal membranes for normalcy and completeness.

- Perform an assessment of the woman in the immediate postpartum period.

- Perform an immediate assessment of the neonate at delivery.

- Explain the procedure and rationale for fundal massage in the postpartum period.

- Identify maternal and neonatal needs during the first hour after birth.

- Discuss family needs and identify advantages of family-centered birth care.

UNIT IV: ADAPTATION IN THE INTRAPARTUM PERIOD

Application of Key Terms

Match the definitions in column two with the key terms in column one.

_____ 1. Apgar score
_____ 2. Atony
_____ 3. Bearing down
_____ 4. Birth attendant
_____ 5. Cotyledon
_____ 6. Crowning
_____ 7. Episiotomy
_____ 8. Introitus

A. Incision into the perineum and vagina during delivery to enlarge the vaginal opening.
B. Lack of normal muscle tone or strength.
C. Segment or subdivision of the uterine surface of the placenta.
D. System of numerical evaluation of neonate's condition at 1 minute and 5 minutes after birth.
E. Distention of the perineum by the largest diameter of the presenting part.
F. Reflex effort on the part of the woman to coordinate activity of the abdominal muscles with the uterine contractions.
G. Vaginal opening.
H. The one who delivers the baby.

Short Answer Exercise of Critical Content

1. During the second stage of labor the fetus descends through the maternal pelvis and the vaginal canal. Specify the two forces that bring about descent at this time.

   a.

   b.

2. Summarize the rationale for using such comfort measures as: cool compresses, ice chips, frozen juice bars or large lollipops during second stage labor.

3. Terri is beginning to bear down with her contractions. She needs instructions in how to push. What instructions would you give Terri so that her pushing style will not cause high intrathoracic pressure and potentially detrimental hemodynamic changes?

NURSING CARE IN NORMAL BIRTH

4. Determine five principles that should be applied in choosing or assisting a woman in assuming a position for delivery.

   a.

   b.

   c.

   d.

   e.

5. List at least three techniques the nurse can use to help the client avoid an episiotomy.

   a.

   b.

   c.

6. Explain why the woman sometimes is asked to pant or breathe through her contractions in second stage.

7. Specify what is meant by a nuchal cord.

8. Susan has delivered her baby and the birth attendant is awaiting the separation of the placenta. List three signs of placental separation.

   a.

   b.

   c.

9. Calculate the one minute Apgar scores for the infants below.

	Baby A	Baby B	Baby C	Baby D	Baby E
Heart Rate	106	Absent	98	120	134
Respiratory Rate	Slow irregular	Slow irregular	Good crying	Good regular	Crying
Muscle tone	Extremities slightly flexed	Flaccid	Moving actively	Slight flexion of extremities	Active movement
Reflex irritability	Grimaces	Grimaces	Crying	No response	Crying
Color	Body pink, extremities blue	Overall pallor and cyanosis	Body pink, hands and feet blue	Body pink, hands and feet blue	Completely pink
Total Score					

10. Describe two interventions for promoting a clear airway in the newborn.

   a.

   b.

11. Describe the procedure for massaging the uterine fundus in the immediate postpartum period.

12. Explain the rationale for massaging the fundus.

13. Relate why fundal massage must be done gently.

14. Identify the two most common causes of postpartum hemorrhage immediately after delivery.

    a.

    b.

15. Sharon comes to the birthing center in active labor and with intact membranes. Eight hours later she delivers a healthy infant with no complications. Thirty minutes after delivery you find that her temperature is 100°F. Explain what you should do.

16. Place an "N" beside the normal findings in fourth stage, and an "A" by those that are abnormal.

    _____ 1. Saturation of two perineal pads in the first hour.
    _____ 2. Rapid pooling of blood under the buttocks.
    _____ 3. Uterus large and soft.
    _____ 4. Fundus midline.
    _____ 5. Slow, intermittent trickle of lochia.
    _____ 6. Small clots in lochia.
    _____ 7. Tissue in lochia.
    _____ 8. Rectal pressure and severe perineal pain.

17. State two observations that would indicate parent-infant attachment is occurring

    a.

    b.

18. List three potential complications of the newborn that must be monitored for during fourth stage.

    a.

    b.

    c.

UNIT IV: ADAPTATION IN THE INTRAPARTUM PERIOD

Multiple Choice Exercise of Critical Content

Circle the most correct answer.

1. Diane, a primigravida, has been in labor since 02:00. She has progressed in labor and is now, eight hours later, 7 cm. How often should you take her vital signs.
    a. Every 30 minutes in low-risk women.
    b. Every 20 minutes in low-risk women.
    c. Every 15 minutes in low-risk women.
    d. Every 5 minutes in low-risk women.

2. Diane becomes very restless and almost argumentative. She throws the bed clothes off and states that she wants to go home. Her actions make you believe she is probably in what phase of labor?
    a. Latent
    b. Transition
    c. First
    d. Second

3. Diane continues in active labor and starts screaming The baby is coming! What is the first thing you as the nurse should do?
    a. Call her birth attendant.
    b. Medicate the patient for pain.
    c. Tell her it is impossible.
    d. Check the perineum.

4. Diane is correct and you have to deliver the baby in the bed. You encourage her to:
    a. Push with all her power.
    b. Cross her legs and pant.
    c. Pant to slow the process.
    d. Hold her breath as long as possible.

5. Diane delivers the head of the infant over an intact perineum. The first thing you do is:
    a. Put Erythromycin ointment in the baby's eyes.
    b. Suction the baby's mouth with deep suction.
    c. Reprimand the mother for pushing the head out and making you deliver the baby.
    d. Feel around the baby's neck for the presence of the umbilical cord.

6. Astrid is in active labor, exhibits fear and anxiety, and is holding her breath during contractions. You encourage her to:

   a. Continue holding her breath during contractions.

   b. Ask all visitors to leave so she can properly concentrate.

   c. Coach her to reestablish appropriate breathing pattern.

   d. Tell her she is doing it wrong and must change her ways.

7. Astrid delivers a full-term male after pushing for an hour. The nurses immediate care of the newborn include:

   a. Assessing infant's respirations, identify infant, keep infant warm.

   b. Applying prophylactic agent to eyes; give Aqua Mephyton, and bathe baby.

   c. Rushing the baby to the nursery while he is suspended by the ankles.

   d. Placing the neonate in a crib and leaving him there until the physician is finished with the mother.

8. During the first hour after birth, Astrid is checked every fifteen minutes. She asks you why you need to keep sticking your hand in her stomach. You would reply:

   a. "This is a good way to check your pain threshold."

   b. "It is always done this way and you must tolerate it."

   c. "It is necessary to do this to make sure the uterus stays firm to decrease bleeding."

   d. "We want to make sure your epidural is wearing off and this is the easiest way to do so."

9. Stacy is 2 hours postdelivery. She is complaining of pain in her abdomen. You palpate the fundus and find it firm and 4 cms above the umbilicus and off to the right. What nursing action is necessary?

   a. Medicate Stacy for abdominal pain.

   b. Encourage her to change her position.

   c. Massage the fundus and try to center it.

   d. Encourage her to empty her bladder.

10. Stacy is unable to void. You try several measures to encourage her to do so. If she is still unable to void what will you do?

    a. Give her some pain medication.

    b. Put her back to bed and try again later.

    c. Obtain an order to catheterize her.

    d. Tell her she needs to continue to try to void.

UNIT IV: ADAPTATION IN THE INTRAPARTUM PERIOD

Matching Exercise of Critical Content

Match the type of laceration with its correct definition.

Type of Laceration	Definition
___ 1. Periclitoral	A. Involving the skin or vaginal mucosa only.
___ 2. Periurethral	B. Extending from the skin and vaginal mucosa into the muscles of the perineum.
___ 3. First degree	C. Extending into the anal sphincter.
___ 4. Second degree	D. Extending through the rectal mucosa into the lumen of the rectum.
___ 5. Third degree	E. A tear near the urethral meatus.
___ 6. Fourth degree	F. A tear near the clitoris.

The interventions below are done to support thermoregulation in the newborn. Rationale for these interventions are noted. Match the interventions with the rationale that best explains them.

Interventions	Rationales
___ 1. Keep delivery room warm.	A. Prevent heat loss by convection
___ 2. Keep delivery room draft free.	B. Prevent heat loss by evaporation
___ 3. Dry baby thoroughly and immediately upon delivery.	C. Prevent heat loss by radiation.
___ 4. Use radiant warmer.	
___ 5. Cover baby with warm blankets.	
___ 6. Place hat on baby.	

True and False Exercise of Critical Content

The following statements require you to assess whether or not they are true or false. If the statement is false rewrite it so that it is correct.

1. The early second stage of labor often is characterized by an increase in the intensity and pace of labor. (True/False).

2. The first part of the second stage allows the nurse to encourage rest, preparation for bearing-down, and reassuring and revitalizing the support person for expulsion. (True/False).

3. The final moments before birth require the utmost attention and concentration on the part of the woman. (True/False).

NURSING CARE IN NORMAL BIRTH

4. Goals of nursing care in the final moments prior to birth include preparing the supplies needed for birth, assisting the birth attendant, and providing physical and emotional support to the woman at the time when her energy levels are often low or depleted. (True/False).

5. During the birth process the nurse moves to the patients feet to be able to assist the birth attendant. (True/False).

6. The nurse must be skilled in neonatal assessment, Apgar scoring, and newborn resuscitation, as well as immediate support of normal adaptations and management of emergencies in the postpartum woman. (True/False).

7. Often the woman experiences deep sleep and relief after she delivers the baby. (True/False).

8. Following the birth, the goal of nursing is to support the physiologic adaptations of the mother and newborn and facilitate the beginning parent-newborn acquaintance process. (True/False).

9. Assessment of maternal and neonatal vital signs and physiologic functioning is essential during the fourth stage of labor. (True/False).

Critical Thinking Exercise

1. Marsha is just fully dilated, but she tells you, "I don't feel like pushing." Explain what nursing interventions you would initiate in response to this comment. Infer the rational behind Marsha's statement and specify the rational behind your interventions.

2. Compare/contrast the "open glottis" pushing technique with traditional methods that use the Valsalva maneuver.

3. Beth has just delivered an 8 pound 8 ounce well developed baby boy after 12 hours of labor. She does not show any interest in the baby. Analyze the situation and explain why Beth may desire limited interaction with her newborn.

CHAPTER 22

Monitoring the At-Risk Fetus

Overview

Maternity care includes a range of technologies and procedures designed to reduce intrapartum risk to the woman and fetus. The nurse must be prepared to care for women and their families so that the level of risk is reduced and emotional needs are met. Discussions about risk reduction procedures must always take into account the relative benefits and risks of more active obstetric management. This chapter focuses on monitoring the at-risk fetus.

Learning Objectives

After studying the material in this chapter, the student will be able to:

- Identify indications for use of electronic fetal monitoring during labor.
- Describe advantages and disadvantages of internal and external fetal monitoring.
- Identify the key elements of fetal heart rate patterns and their normal range.
- Discuss the nurse's role in the application electronic fetal monitoring and interpretation of its data.
- Describe the advantages and disadvantages of fetal scalp sampling and fetal scalp stimulation.
- Explain the kind of information obtained from fetal scalp sampling and scalp stimulation.
- Describe the new technologies and the kinds of information obtained.

MONITORING THE AT-RISK FETUS

APPLICATION OF KEY TERMS

Match the definitions in column two with the key terms in column one.

_____ 1. Baseline fetal heart rate
_____ 2. Doppler velocimetry
_____ 3. Fetal distress
_____ 4. Fetal stress
_____ 5. Intrauterine pressure catheter
_____ 6. Long-term variability
_____ 7. Short-term variability
_____ 8. Sinusoidal pattern
_____ 9. Spiral electrode
_____ 10. Tokodynamometer

A. Average fetal heart rate within a 10-minute interval in the absence of or between contractions.

B. A term for the nonspecific biologic responses in the fetus elicited by adverse external influences.

C. A state of physiologic decompensation or compromise in the fetus caused by a lack of oxygen and nutrients.

D. A pressure-sensing instrument that records the relative strength of uterine contractions.

E. Cyclic variations of 6 to 10 bpm amplitude around the baseline heart rate in 3 to 10 cycles per minute.

F. A wire that is gently twisted beneath the fetal scalp while inutero; used to monitor FHT.

G. Catheter inserted into the uterus after the membranes are ruptured to monitor contractions.

H. A noninvasive technique that permits measurement of blood flow velocity in the fetal aorta and umbilical artery.

I. Wavelike changes in the fetal heart tracing that can only be detected with internal monitoring.

J. An unusual FHR a pattern that shows uniform wavelike long-term variability of 5 to 15 bpm every 3 to 5 minutes, minimal or absent beat-to-beat variability, and absence of specific responses to uterine contractions.

Short Answer Exercise of Critical Content

1. For the following scenarios, identify whether external (E) or internal (I) electronic fetal monitors should be used and which of the following problems, if any, exist.

PROBLEMS:

Bradycardia

Tachycardia

Long-term variability (specify degree)

Poor beat-to-beat variability

Sinusoidal pattern.

Late deceleration

Variable deceleration

Dysrhythmia

No evident FHR problems

  a. FHR 120-132 with good beat-to-beat variability and no periodic changes. Mother is post-term and slightly hypertensive. (E/I).

b. FHR 155-170 with beat-to-beat variability decreasing. (E/I).

c. FHR 125-128 with no periodic changes. (E/I).

d. FHR 140-160 with occasional 175 upon fetal movement and uniform drop to 130 at peak of contraction. (E/I).

e. FHR 130-140 with differing shape and timing of decreases to 90 for 30 to 50 seconds. (E/I).

2. There are three major patterns of decelerations. Complete the following chart with the identified causes, characteristics, and clinical significance.

Type	Cause	Characteristics	Clinical Significance
Early deceleration			
Late deceleration			
Variable deceleration			

3. List the interventions the nurse must take to maximize uteroplacental perfusion in the case of signs of fetal distress.

   a.

   b.

   c.

   d.

   e.

   f.

MONITORING THE AT-RISK FETUS

Multiple Choice Exercise of Critical Content

Circle the most correct answer.

1. Leslie is in active labor and you note persistent early decelerations on the fetal monitoring strip. What would be the most appropriate nursing action?
   a. Do nothing, the pattern is benign.
   b. Perform a vaginal examination to determine if the cord has prolapsed.
   c. Stay with the woman and observe what happens with the next contraction.
   d. Turn the woman to her left side and start administering oxygen.

2. While working with Leslie, you observe the monitor and should not which of the following factors?
   a. Baseline fetal heart rate.
   b. Accelerations and decelerations of the fetal heart rate.
   c. Relationship of fetal heart rate to uterine contractions.
   d. All of the above are true observations.

3. Leslie asks you what the most common deceleration pattern is. Your response would be:
   a. Variable decelerations.
   b. Early decelerations.
   c. Bradycardia.
   d. Late decelerations.

4. Audrey is having early decelerations. These are most often caused by:
   a. The mother's position.
   b. Uteroplacental insufficiency.
   c. Compression of the fetal head.
   d. Compression of the umbilical cord.

5. Kristen is experiencing late decelerations. You have turned her to her left side and started O_2. The fetal heart rate is slow to respond. You call for assistance and flip her to her right side. The late deceleration are probably due to:
   a. Hypotension.
   b. Compression of the fetal head.
   c. Uteroplacental insufficiency.
   d. Compression of the umbilical cord.

True and False Exercise of Critical Content

The following statements require you to assess whether or not they are true or false. If the statement is false, rewrite it so that it is correct.

1. The maternity nurse must have a thorough understanding of fetal distress and the implications for nursing care when fetal distress is suspected. (True/False).

2. The nurse makes the decisions when abnormal patterns are identified and shields the woman until the problem is resolved. (True/False).

3. The need for fetal scalp sampling reduces the woman's control over the process of labor. (True/False).

4. With fetal scalp stimulation the fetal heart rate should decelerate. (True/False).

5. Cordocentesis or percutaneous umbilical cord blood sampling is the transabdominal needle aspiration of umbilical cord blood for the analysis of fetal blood gas and acid-based parameters. (True/False).

MONITORING THE AT-RISK FETUS

Critical Thinking Exercise

1. Analyze the positive and negative aspects seen from application of electronic fetal monitors.

2. Compare and contrast external versus internal electronic fetal monitoring.

3. Danielle refused EFM when meconium-stained fluid was detected. Evaluate her reason(s) for refusing EFM. Formulate a plan to explain the rational for the use of EFM.

CHAPTER 23

Modifying Labor Patterns and Mode of Delivery

Overview

Some women require interventions to modify a less than optimal labor pattern or a difficult labor. When this occurs, nursing care is focused on explaining the procedures, clarifying questions the woman or family may have, maintaining maternal and fetal physiologic status, and providing emotional and physical support. To allow for the safest, most satisfying birth experience possible, the nurse must be able to balance to technologic approach to care with intensive emotional support.

Learning Objectives

After studying the material in this chapter, the student will be able to:

- Distinguish between induction and augmentation of labor and identify the common modes of each.

- Discuss nursing responsibilities during and after amniotomy.

- List major precautions to be considered when infusing oxytocin.

- Identify indications for and precautions taken during forceps applications.

- State the indications for cesarean birth.

- Discuss nursing responsibilities in caring for the woman and her family before, during, and after cesarean birth.

- Identify contraindications and necessary precautions for a trial of labor and vaginal birth after cesarean delivery.

- Explain nursing responsibilities when uterine hyperstimulation is identified during augmentation or induction of labor.

MODIFYING LABOR PATTERNS AND MODE OF DELIVERY

Application of Key Terms

Match the definitions in column two with the key terms in column one.

_____ 1. Amniotomy
_____ 2. Augmentation of labor
_____ 3. Bishop score
_____ 4. Cervical ripening
_____ 5. Cord prolapse
_____ 6. Forceps
_____ 7. Induction of labor
_____ 8. Intrauterine fetal resuscitation
_____ 9. Laminaria
_____ 10. Macrosomia
_____ 11. Malpresentation
_____ 12. Meconium
_____ 13. Oxytocin
_____ 14. Prostaglandin E_2 gel
_____ 15. Stripping membranes
_____ 16. Tetanic contractions
_____ 17. Tocolysis
_____ 18. Version

A. Genus of moisture-absorbing seaweed used to dilate the cervix before elective abortion.
B. Two-bladed instrument used to assist delivery of the fetus after the cervix is fully dilated and the fetal head is engaged.
C. Artificial rupture of the amniotic sac or bag of waters.
D. Fecal material discharged by the newborn.
E. Abnormally long uterine contraction, lasting more than 70 seconds.
F. Unusually large baby.
G. Obstetric emergency in which the umbilical cord descends into or through the cervix ahead of the presenting fetal part.
H. Faulty or abnormal fetal presentation.
I. Drug used to stimulate uterine contractions to assist childbirth and prevent postdelivery hemorrhage.
J. Drug that diminishes the force of uterine contractions.
K. Manipulation to alter presentation of the fetus.
L. A system that provides a score assessing cervical dilatation, effacement, consistency, and position as well as fetal station.
M. The digital separation of the amniotic membranes from the wall of the lower uterine segment near the cervix.
N. Causes effacement and softening of the cervix; used for cervical ripening.
O. The process of promoting more effective uterine contractions when labor has already begun but is dysfunctional or has stopped completely.
P. Changes that normally occur in late pregnancy that prepare the cervix for labor.
Q. Use of oxytocin to cause contractions that begin labor.
R. The use of a tocolytic drug in cases of fetal distress when uterine activity is contributing to fetal hypoxia.

Short Answer Exercise of Critical Content

1. At 42 weeks gestation, Wanda, gravida 2 para 1, is admitted to labor and delivery for labor induction. Evaluate why induction of labor would be indicated for Wanda.

2. Wanda's birth attendant decides to initiate labor by performing an amniotomy. Explain the procedure to Wanda.

3. Nursing interventions prior to the amniotomy include:

   a.

   b.

   c.

4. After the amniotomy nursing interventions would include:

   a.

   b.

   c.

   d.

   e.

5. Four hours later Wanda's contractions are occurring irregularly with mild intensity. The birth attendant writes orders to augment Wanda's contractions with oxytocin infusion. List 5 nursing assessments during augmentation.

   a.

   b.

   c.

   d.

   e.

6. After six hours of active labor, Sue, gravida 1, para 0, is informed of the possibility of a cesarean delivery because of persistent late decelerations. Plan pre-operative teaching interventions to assist Sue and her husband prepare for an emergency cesarean.

MODIFYING LABOR PATTERNS AND MODE OF DELIVERY

7. Identify how the nursing staff can promote a family-centered birth experience for Sue and her husband.

8. A low-segment cesarean section with a pfannenstiel incision is performed. Describe anatomically where Sue's incisions are located.

9. Would Sue be a candidate for a vaginal birth after cesarean (VBAC) with a future pregnancy? Under what conditions?

10. Mary's efforts to push the baby out have become ineffective because she is exhausted. The birth attendant decides it is time to deliver the baby with outlet forceps. Define outlet forceps.

Multiple Choice Exercise of Critical Content

Circle the most correct answer.

1. Debra's membranes rupture suddenly at the end of a contraction. Your first nursing action would be to:
    a. Assess fetal heart rate.
    b. Change the bed to enhance Debra's comfort.
    c. Instruct Debra to push.
    d. Notify the birth attendant immediately.

2. After Debra's membranes rupture her contractions decrease in frequency and intensity. The birth attendant orders oxytocin to be given. You will watch Debra closely for:
    a. Decreased uterine activity.
    b. Uterine hyperstimulation.
    c. Thirst associated with increased temperature.
    d. Need to repeat rupture of membranes.

3. Abby's baby is in a breech position. The birth attendant is planning external podalic version. You know this is being done because:
   a. The presenting part is not engaged in the pelvis.
   b. Ultrasound evaluation has located the placenta and ruled out multiple gestation.
   c. The maternal abdominal wall is thin, permitting accurate palpation.
   d. All of the above are required conditions.

4. The birth attendant determines Judy is unable to push the infant out due to a tight fetopelvic fit and plans a low forcep delivery. Criteria for low forcep delivery include:
   a. The fetal head is visible at the vaginal introitus.
   b. The fetal head is at the level of the ischial spines and engaged.
   c. The leading point of the fetal skull is at or greater than +2 station.
   d. An emergency cesarean delivery is unavailable.

5. Shantrice, gravida 2, para 1, is undergoing trial labor because she is VBAC. What previous condition that lead to the first cesarean delivery would prevent her from delivering vaginally this time?
   a. Low-segment uterine incision with previous cesarean.
   b. The pervious section was done for CPD.
   c. Availability of emergency surgical facilities.
   d. The previous section was done for fetal distress.

True and False Exercise of Critical Content

The following statements require you to assess whether or not they are true or false. If the statement is false, rewrite it so that it is correct.

1. The nurse does not have a role in the augmentation or induction of labor. (True/False).

2. If complications arise during an induction, the nurse provides immediate supportive care and must be prepared to assist the birth attendant with diagnostic procedures during an emergency delivery. (True/False).

3. When complications arise that require the birth attendant to modify the normal mode of vaginal delivery, the nurse withdraws from participation. (True/False).

MODIFYING LABOR PATTERNS AND MODE OF DELIVERY

4. During complications and emergencies, a goal of nursing care is to facilitate a family-centered birth experience, regardless of the mode of delivery. (True/False).

Critical Thinking Exercise

1. LaTonya is at 42 weeks gestation and is scheduled for insertion of prostaglandin gel for cervical ripening at 4:30 pm and induction with oxytocin at 6:30 am the next morning. Explain the appropriate nursing care for the two procedures.

2. Brenda is scheduled for an emergency cesarean delivery. Develop a plan to provide preoperative preparation, teaching, and emotional support prior to the cesarean surgery.

3. Determine how the nurse can promote family-centered care in the event of an unscheduled cesarean delivery that requires administration of a general anesthetic.

CHAPTER 24

Managing Pain During the Intrapartum and Postpartum Periods

Overview

Each woman experiences the physical sensations of labor differently. Discomfort, pain, and pressure are words often used to describe sensations accompanying childbirth. Many nurses have been educated to avoid the use of the word pain in relation to contractions. Most nurses believe that some degree of pain is experienced by most women during labor and birth, even though the pain varies widely in nature, extent, and location. Although minor discomforts are common in the immediate postpartum period, unrelieved pain that interferes with rest and sleep or the ability to perform activities of daily living requires prompt alleviation. This chapter reviews the causes of discomfort or pain experienced during childbirth and during postpartum period and discusses pharmacologic methods used to control these sensations.

Learning Objectives

After studying the material in this chapter, the student will be able to:

- Discuss the causes of pain in childbirth.
- Outline the adverse effects of pain on maternal and fetal well-being.
- Explain the behavioral cues of pain in the woman during labor and birth.
- Describe common verbal indicators of pain during childbirth.
- Identify the most common types of obstetric analgesia and anesthesia.
- List advantages and disadvantages of obstetric analgesia and anesthesia.
- Describe nursing responsibilities during administration of analgesia or anesthesia.
- List major complications of obstetric analgesia and anesthesia.

MANAGING PAIN DURING THE INTRAPARTUM AND POSTPARTUM PERIODS 147

Application of Key Terms

Match the definitions in column two with the key terms in column one.

_____ 1. Analgesia

_____ 2. Anesthesia

_____ 3. General anesthesia

_____ 4. Local anesthesia

_____ 5. Regional anesthesia

A. Partial or complete loss of sensation with or without loss of consciousness.

B. Pharmacologic pain relief measures that block sensory nerve pathways along large sensory nerves from an organ and surrounding tissue, providing loss of sensation in that organ and the surrounding area.

C. The absence or decreased awareness of pain without loss of consciousness.

D. Pharmacologic pain relief measures that block sensory nerve pathways at the organ level, producing loss of sensation in that organ only.

E. Pharmacologic pain relief measures that produce progressive central nervous system depression, loss of consciousness, and thus loss of sensation from the entire body.

Short Answer Exercise of Critical Content

1. Provide the reason for administering IV medication at the beginning of a contraction.

2. Maternal vital signs and fetal heart rate should be assessed and recorded before and shortly after administration of pain medication because a major side effect is:

3. When receiving an epidural, a client may develop hypotension. An early sign of developing hypotension is sudden:

4. In order to elevate blood pressure by relieving pressure on the vena cava, the pregnant woman should be placed in what position?

5. Following administration of anesthesia, why must the mother be monitored for urinary retention?

6. A common side effect of a paracervical block the nurse should be aware of is what?

UNIT IV: ADAPTATION IN THE INTRAPARTUM PERIOD

7. In order to counteract potential hypotension, what should precede epidural anesthesia?

8. List two nursing measures that would help decrease the occurrence of postspinal headache.

9. Indicate the reason why delivery must occur within 5 to 7 minutes following administration of inhalation anesthetics.

10. List the common maternal problems related to general anesthesia.

Multiple Choice Exercise of Critical Content

Circle the most correct answer.

1. Betty has been determined to be in active labor and has requested epidural anesthesia. The nurse prepares the patient by:
   a. Sitting the patient up on the side of the bed.
   b. Placing the patient in a prone position.
   c. Having the patient stand and lean over the bed.
   d. Placing the patient in a trendelenburg position.

2. Betty experiences warmth and tingling of her legs with the test dose without paralysis, sensory impairment, or signs of intravascular injection. You know that this indicates:
   a. An abnormality that requires immediate resuscitation.
   b. The needle has been properly positioned in the epidural space.
   c. Betty will have rapid perineal anesthesia and loss of contractions.
   d. Betty will experience infection at the injection site.

3. Because of large volumes of IV fluids and the blocked bladder sensations Betty will need to be assessed how often for bladder distention?
   a. Every 2 hours.
   b. Every hour.
   c. Every 30 minutes.
   d. Every 15 minutes.

4. Women who receive Duramorph epidurals for cesarean delivery need to be closely monitored for:

   a. Respiratory distress.

   b. Persistent nausea and vomiting.

   c. Urinary retention.

   d. All of the above.

5. Jennifer is experiencing post-surgical pain after administration of a morphine epidural. Which drug would the anesthesiologist most likely order?

   a. Demerol 25 mg IM.

   b. Morphine 10 mg IV.

   c. Toradol 30 mg IM.

   d. Demerol 50 mg IV.

Match Exercise of Critical Content

Match the type of anesthesia in column 2 with the correct description in column 1.

	Description	Anesthesia
___	1. Anesthetic is introduced into cerebrospinal fluid.	A. Paracervical
___	2. Anesthetic is inhaled or given IV.	B. Lumbar epidural
___	3. Purpose is to anesthetize the uterus.	C. Caudal epidural
___	4. Anesthesia inserted at the base of spine.	D. Spinal (subarachnoid)
___	5. Anesthesia is introduced near, but not through, the dura.	E. General

True and False Exercise of Critical Content

The following statements rquire you to assess whether or not they are true or false. If the statement is false, rewrite it so that it is correct.

1. Because nurses are generally responsible for the promotion and administration of analgesics, they must have a comprehensive knowledge regarding these agents, including the normal dosages, indications and contraindications for use, drug precautions, and effective antidotes to adverse reactions. (True/False).

2. Once analgesics are administered, the nurse monitors maternal well-being and continues to provide nonpharmacologic comfort measures to enhance their effectiveness. (True/False).

3. Nurses play a central role in the safe use of anesthetic agents during labor and delivery. (True/False).

4. When general anesthesia is used, there is no bonding between the infant and parents. (True/False).

5. Advances in pain control permit the woman who has experienced an operative delivery to assume self-care and infant care activities at an earlier stage in the postbirth period. (True/False).

Critical Thinking Exercise

1. Lina has reached transition and is demanding some relief from her "pain". Explain why is inadvisable to administer analgesia during the transition stage of labor. Recommend other methods of "pain" control during this stage.

2. Monica has received a narcotic epidural. Specify what the nurse's responsibilities are in the first 24 hours postpartum after administration of a narcotic epidural.

3. Critique the advantages and disadvantages of general anesthesia for operative delivery.

CHAPTER 25

Nursing Care of the At-Risk family in the Perinatal Period

Overview

When complications arise during the perinatal period, they may have devastating effects for the woman and her fetus or newborn. The family is thrust into a situation for which they may not be well prepared and over which they have little control. Outcomes are not predictable, and survival may be uncertain at time. This chapter first discusses the concept of family crisis and explores current theories regarding perinatal loss, the grieving process, and grief work.

Learning Objectives

After studying the material in this chapter, the student will be able to:

- Describe family responses to major perinatal complications.

- Identify factors that affect how women and their families respond to complications.

- Describe phases of the grieving process when complications arise during the perinatal period.

- Identify selected nursing diagnoses for the at-risk family that may occur during the perinatal period.

- Identify common elements in nursing care of the individual and family when complications occur during the perinatal period.

- Explain the importance of a family-centered approach to high-risk perinatal care.

- Describe ways in which family-centered care can be implemented for women and families experiencing perinatal complications.

- Discuss nursing assessment of the high-risk family in terms of crisis theory.

- Describe phases of the grieving process in parents of high-risk or sick neonates.

- List significant signs of potential parenting disorders that may be observed in the assessment of parents of a high-risk or sick neonate.

Application of Key Terms

Match the definitions in column two with the key terms in column one.

_____ 1. Adaptation

_____ 2. Crisis

_____ 3. Empathy

_____ 4. Grief process

_____ 5. Grief work

_____ 6. Intrauterine fetal demise

_____ 7. Perinatal period

A. Objective awareness or recognition of another person's feelings.

B. Period from the 28th week of gestation through the 28th day after birth.

C. Process of responding to internal or environmental stimuli.

D. Sudden change in condition; a turning point during which disorganization occurs because normal coping mechanisms fail.

E. Painful withdrawal of attachment to a lost object or wish during which memories that bind the individual are lost.

F. Fetal death after 20 weeks gestation and the fetus may be retained for some time.

G. Goals include acceptance of the loss, experience the pain of grief, adjust to the environment in which the loss has occurred, and reinvest the energy expended to restore one's life.

Short Answer Exercise of Critical Content

1. List the three factors that are crucial in the resolution of a potential crisis.

    a.

    b.

    c.

2. When problems are diagnosed during the perinatal period, a grief response ensues in parents and close family members. List the stages of grief in their order of occurrence.

   a.

   b.

   c.

   d.

   e.

3. One of the most common treatments recommended for preterm labor, incompetent cervix, or placenta previa is:

4. List the feelings hospitalized high-risk women often express.

   a.

   b.

   c.

   d.

Multiple Choice Exercise of Critical Content

Circle the most correct answer.

1. Belinda delivered at 30 weeks gestation and her baby is in the neonatal intensive care unit. It is best that Belinda and Gene, her husband, be:
   a. Discouraged from visiting the neonate because it will probably die.
   b. Given the opportunity to visually or physically make contact to sense the neonate is real.
   c. Told about all of the defects the baby has.
   d. Not allowed to visit the neonate together because policy allows only one visitor at a time.

2. Belinda and Gene's baby does survive and after 8 months is ready for discharge. The goals of discharge teaching include:

   a. Telling the parents to go home and everything will be alright.

   b. Offering to call them no sooner than next month to remind them of a doctor's appointment.

   c. Decreasing the stress of the transition to home by teaching them and having them practice techniques.

   d. Blaming them for the problems the baby has experienced and will have the rest of it life.

3. Tammy went to her health care providers office alone, and reported she had not felt any fetal movement for the past two days. IUFD was confirmed with ultrasound. The nurse should help Tammy by doing all except:

   a. Begin bereavement interventions.

   b. Accompany Tammy to the hospital for induction.

   c. Send her home to collect her belongings.

   d. Call the labor unit to update Tammy's prenatal records.

True and False Exercise of Critical Content

The following statements require you to assess whether or not they are true or false. if the statement is false, rewrite it so that it is correct.

1. Although individual responses to the development of perinatal complications vary, most family members demonstrate a pattern of grieving that has fairly predictable stages. (True/False).

2. Families usually display no clues to identify the stage of the grieving process, therefore it is impossible to initiate appropriate nursing interventions. (True/False).

3. The most profound loss is intrapartum death; this type of loss is also difficult for the health care team. (True/False).

NURSING CARE OF THE AT-RISK FAMILY IN THE PERINATAL PERIOD

Critical Thinking Exercise

1. Mirenda gave birth to a neonate with multiple anomalies. Evaluate your own reactions and feelings. Plan ways to allow Mirenda to view the neonate and assist her to work through her own feelings.

2. Claudia's newborn has been in the intensive care unit for three days. Claudia has not visited nor called the unit. Today she visits for the first time and is hostile towards and displays distrust of the staff. Determine if Claudia is displaying signs of maladaptive responses. Formulate specific nursing interventions you can implement to support Claudia and help her through the grief process.

CHAPTER 26

Intrapartum Complications

Overview

When complications arise in the intrapartum period, they may develop rapidly and can have devastating effects on the well-being of the woman, fetus, or neonate. The nurse must identify intrapartum problems and intervene in a timely manner to reduce or limit detrimental effects on the woman and fetus. Although many women with obstetric or medical complications may be transported to high-risk perinatal centers, all labor and delivery nurses must possess the knowledge and skills required to deal with obstetric emergencies. This chapter focuses on the major complications that occur during the intrapartum period and discusses appropriate medical and nursing management of the high-risk intrapartum woman.

Learning Objectives

After studying the material in this chapter, the student will be able to:

- Compare and contrast the common causes, signs, and symptoms of placenta previa and abruptio placentae.

- Outline medical and nursing care for the woman when placenta previa or abruptio placentae complicates the intrapartum period.

- Compare and contrast the causes, signs, and symptoms of oligohydramnios and polyhydramnios.

- Outline the medical and nursing care when oligohydramnios or polyhydramnios complicates the intrapartum period.

- Identify risks of umbilical cord prolapse to the woman and fetus.

- Discuss the required emergency nursing interventions when umbilical cord prolapse occurs.

- Describe the four major causes of labor dystocia.

- Outline the medical and nursing care for the woman with labor dystocia due to the four causes.

- Compare and contrast the causes, signs, and symptoms of hypovolemic and septic shock.

- Outline nursing responsibilities in the treatment of hypovolemic shock.

- Discuss disseminated intravascular coagulopathy in terms of etiology, diagnosis, and medical and nursing care.

- Identify common causes, signs, and symptoms for uterine rupture.

- Outline nursing responsibilities in the care of the woman with uterine rupture.

- Identify common causes, signs, and symptoms for amniotic fluid embolus.

- Outline nursing responsibilities in the care of the woman with amniotic fluid embolus.

INTRAPARTUM COMPLICATIONS

Application of Key Terms

Match the definitions in column two with the key terms in column one.

    1. Abruptio placentae
    2. Bicornuate uterus
    3. Chorioamnionitis
    4. Cor pulmonale
    5. Disseminated intravascular coagulopathy
    6. Dystocia
    7. Endotoxin
    8. Exsanguination
    9. Hypotonic labor
  10. Hypertonic labor
  11. Placenta previa
  12. Retraction ring
  13. Shock
  14. Vasa praevia
  15. Velamentous insertion

A. A placenta that is implanted in the lower uterine segment.

B. Anomaly of insertion of the umbilical cord in which the umbilical blood vessels traverse the lower uterine segment and present at delivery in advance of the head.

C. A pathologic form of coagulation, diffuse throughout the body, in which certain clotting factors are consumed to the extent that generalized bleeding occurs.

D. Complete or partial separation of the normally implanted placenta from the uterine wall.

E. Inflammation of the chorion and amnion.

F. Difficult labor resulting from fetal or maternal causes.

G. Toxin confined within bacteria and freed when the bacteria are broken down.

H. Insertion of the umbilical cord where the blood vessels leave the placenta, course between the amnion and chorion, and unite to form the umbilical cord at some distance from the edge of the placenta.

I. Extensive, severe blood loss that is so extreme that it is incompatible with life.

J. Failure of the uterine muscles to contract and retract with normal strength and frequency.

K. Physiologic area of constriction at the junction of the upper, or contracting, portion and the lower, or dilating, portion of the uterus.

L. Uterus in which the fundus is divided into two parts.

M. State of greater than normal muscle tension.

N. Dilation and failure of the right side of the heart due to pulmonary embolism.

O. The body's response to life-threatening physiologic conditions.

Short Answer Exercise of Critical Content

1. List five reasons for maternal transport to a tertiary center for care.

   a.

   b.

   c.

   d.

   e.

2. Identify three causes of chorioamnionitis.

   a.

   b.

   c.

3. List five of the most commonly occurring congenital problems associated with polyhydramnios.

   a.

   b.

   c.

   d.

   e.

INTRAPARTUM COMPLICATIONS

4. Common predisposing factors for umbilical cord prolapse would include:

   a.

   b.

   c.

   d.

5. Women with multifetal gestation are frequently candidates for what method of delivery? Why?

6. Renee is 43 weeks gestation and the health care provider is watching her closely. You know that establishing a diagnosis of fetal postmaturity syndrome requires careful prenatal testing and evaluation of the fetus, including:

   a.

   b.

   c.

   d.

   e.

UNIT IV: ADAPTATION IN THE INTRAPARTUM PERIOD

7. Many factors contribute to the quality of labor. Identify four factors that are of primary importance in determining whether progress is made.

   a.

   b.

   c.

   d.

8. Breech presentations are a common cause of dystocia and often are indications for cesarean deliveries. Why?

9. The criteria for diagnosing a precipitous labor would be:

10. Louisa is in labor and has been experiencing tetanic contractions. Suddenly she experiences intense, sharp, tearing pain and all contractions stop. You would expect what has just happened?

11. Etiologic and Predisposing factors of DIC include what events?

   a.

   b.

   c.

   d.

   e.

INTRAPARTUM COMPLICATIONS

12. Anita is receiving oxytocin augmentation for her labor. She is very restless and has been coughing up frothy pink sputum. You notify the health care provider immediately because you know this could be a premonitary sign of what?

Multiple Choice Exercise of Critical Content

Circle the most correct answer.

1. Jeanette is experiencing hyperactive labor. Signs and symptoms of hyperactive labor include all of the following *except*:
   a. Contractions every two minutes, lasting 90 seconds.
   b. Rapid progressive cervical dilatation.
   c. A prolonged latent phase.
   d. Severe discomfort with mild contractions.

2. Melanie, 20 years old, a primigravida is admitted at term to the labor unit. She has a moderate amount of dark vaginal bleeding and no uterine contractions. Fetal heart rate is 145 to 150. Your first nursing action would be to:
   a. Prepare for speculum examination by the birth attendant.
   b. Do a vaginal examination to determine cervical dilatation.
   c. Prepare to give Melanie a soap-suds enema.
   d. Prepare to send Melanie back home because she is not in active labor.

3. After Melanie is examined she experiences a board like abdomen. Melanie most likely is experiencing:
   a. Abruptio placentae.
   b. Placenta previa.
   c. Normal labor.
   d. Placenta accreta.

4. Dina is diagnosed with a Frank breech position. Frank breech is defined as the position in which:
   a. The normal attitude of flexion is maintained and the fetus sits tailor-fashion in the pelvis.
   b. One foot presents at the cervix.
   c. The knees are extended, the thighs are flexed, and the buttocks present.
   d. Both feet present at the cervix.

5. Dina's pelvis is considered adequate for vaginal delivery. Because of the breech presentation she might experience:

   a. A greater amount of bloody show during labor.

   b. Slower labor progress than normal.

   c. More intense labor contractions.

   d. A more rapid labor than normal.

6. In the event of an impending precipitous delivery, the nurse should take what action?

   a. Hold the head of the fetus back until the birth attendant arrives.

   b. Give the patient ether to relax her.

   c. Remain with the patient to coach and assist her.

   d. Leave her room to call the birth attendant.

7. While performing a vaginal examination, you discover a glistening white cord protruding from the vagina. Your first nursing action would be to:

   a. Leave the patients room to place an emergency call to the birth attendant.

   b. Start administering oxygen by mask at 3L and assess the mother's vital signs.

   c. Place sterile 4x4s over the cord and moisten them with sterile normal saline.

   d. Apply manual pressure to presenting part and put patient into Trendelenburg or knee-chest position.

8. In the case of a prolapsed cord, you know your action was effective if you observe:

   a. The mother does not develop an infection.

   b. There is no excessive vaginal bleeding.

   c. The fetal heart tones remain at previous baseline level.

   d. The mother's vital signs remain at her normal range.

Matching Exercise of Critical Content

Match the following symptoms with the appropriate condition.

SYMPTOM:	CONDITION:
1. Painless vaginal bleeding.	A. Placenta previa
2. Uterine pain.	B. Abruptio placentae
3. Soft uterus.	
4. Hemorrhage may be concealed.	
5. Floating presenting part.	
6. Rigid, boardlike abdomen.	
7. Associated with cocaine use.	

INTRAPARTUM COMPLICATIONS

True and False Exercise of Critical Content

The following statements require you to assess whether or not they are true or false. If the statement is false, rewrite it so that it is correct.

1. Perinatal regionalization has made it possible to transport women with intrapartum complications when special treatment is required. (True/False).

2. Medical diagnosis alone, provides the nurse with a systematic method of identifying intrapartum problems and planning appropriate care. (True.False).

3. Complications involving the placenta can result in fetal distress or death and maternal life-threatening hemorrhage. (True/False).

4. Regardless of the setting, the maternity nurse must be prepared to initiate emergency measures to support the woman and fetus until medical help arrives. (True/False).

5. When infection of the fetal membranes occurs, there is no threat to maternal well-being. (True/False).

6. When abnormalities of the umbilical cord occur, the fetus is at greater risk for abnormalities, exsanguination, and fetal distress. (True/False).

7. When fetal problems complicate the intrapartum period, the focus of nursing care generally is on assessment of maternal well-being. (True/False).

8. Dystocia usually causes anxiety, pain, and fatigue for the woman. (True/False).

9. DIC is characterized by generation of increased prothrombin, platelets, and other coagulation factors that cause widespread formation of thrombi throughout the microvasculature. (True/False).

10. Events leading to cardiopulmonary collapse are initial pulmonary hypertension, corpulmonale, reduced left atrial pressure, reduced carbon dioxide, and systemic hypotension. (True/False)

Critical Thinking Exercise

1. Chantal is in active labor. The FHR has been 136 to 150. Suddenly you see dips in the FHR to 100 with elevations to 165. Specify signs and symptoms of the FHR pattern that would suggest umbilical cord compression.

2. Wendy has been in prolonged labor for 36 hours. Develop a nursing care plan to assist Wendy.

3. Tara delivered her baby in the taxi on her way to the birthing center. Determine your primary nursing responsibilities to assist Tara when she arrives.

4. Dorothy is experiencing excessive vaginal bleeding following delivery. Assess Dorothy for signs and symptoms that would indicate that she is experiencing hypovolemic shock or DIC.

CHAPTER 27

Perinatal High-Risk Challenges

Overview

Some women begin pregnancy with underlying medical problems that may compromise maternal, fetal, and neonatal well-being. Others develop significant obstetric complications that alter the subsequent course and outcome of the childbearing process. These problems require active, ongoing medical and nursing management throughout the gestational period, during childbirth, and the immediate post-partum period. This chapter describes major complications that occur during the perinatal period.

Learning Objectives

After studying the material in this chapter, the student will be able to:

- List predisposing factors associated with preterm labor and birth.

- Compare and contrast tocolytics currently used in the treatment of preterm labor in terms of dosages, route of administration, side affects, adverse reactions, and nursing implications.

- Discuss fetal and neonatal complications related to preterm premature rupture of membranes.

- Outline the medical management and nursing care for the woman with preterm premature rupture of membranes.

- Discuss current theories regarding the etiology of pregnancy-induced hypertension.

- Outline the classic signs and symptoms of pregnancy-induced hypertension.

- Outline the medical management and nursing care of the woman with pregnancy-induced hypertension.

- Define eclampsia and describe the major nursing care when eclamptic seizures occur.

- Compare and contrast the etiology and clinical signs and symptoms of disseminated intravascular coagulopathy and HELLP syndrome.

- Describe pregnancy changes that predispose the woman to the development of carbohydrate intolerance and diabetes.

- Identify maternal, fetal, and neonatal risks when diabetes complicates pregnancy.

- Define diabetic ketoacidosis, its medical treatment, and appropriate nursing care.

- Describe signs and symptoms of hypoglycemia and the nurse's role in its treatment.

- Outline major aspects of nursing and medical management when cardiac disease complicates pregnancy.

Application of Key Terms

Match the definitions in column two with the key terms in column one.

____ 1. Disseminated intravascular coagulopathy
____ 2. Eclampsia
____ 3. Ketoacidosis
____ 4. Neuropathy
____ 5. Petechiae
____ 6. Plasma oncotic pressure
____ 7. Preeclampsia
____ 8. Pregnancy-induced hypertension
____ 9. Premature rupture of membranes
____ 10. Preterm labor
____ 11. Retinopathy
____ 12. Scotoma
____ 13. Tocolytic

A. Small, purplish hemorrhagic spots on the skin.
B. Drug that diminishes the force of uterine contractions.
C. Abnormal condition characterized by inflammation and degeneration of peripheral nerves.
D. Disorder of pregnancy or the postpartum period characterized by hypertension, edema, and proteinuria.
E. Labor that occurs before the 37th week of gestation.
F. Toxemia of pregnancy accompanied by high blood pressure, albuminuria, oliguria, tonic and clonic convulsions, and coma; may occur before, during, or after childbirth.
G. Acidosis accompanied by excessive ketones in the body and resulting from faulty carbohydrate metabolism.
H. Rupture of the amniotic sac before the onset of uterine contractions.
I. A pathologic form of coagulation, diffuse throughout the body, in which certain clotting factors are consumed to the extent that generalized bleeding occurs.
J. Blind spot in the visual field.
K. Disorder of the retina associated with diabetes, hypertension, and toxemia of pregnancy.
L. A hypertensive disorder unique to pregnancy.
M. Associated with a cause of pulmonary edema.

Short Answer Exercise of Critical Content

1. Cite five obstetric risk factors associated with preterm labor.

    a.

    b.

    c.

    d.

    e.

PERINATAL HIGH-RISK CHALLENGES

2. Determine the diagnostic criteria for preterm labor.

3. The oldest and simplest treatment for preterm labor include _____ and _____.

4. Carla has been diagnosed with preterm labor at 25 weeks gestation. She is being treated with 2.5 mg Brethine every 4 hours. What side effects should she be told to expect?

5. List four factors that affect the fetal outcome with premature rupture of membranes.

   a.

   b.

   c.

   d.

6. Nursing care for a patient with premature rupture of membranes includes:

   a.

   b.

   c.

   d.

   e.

7. List six risk factors for developing PIH.

   a.

   b.

   c.

   d.

   e.

   f.

8. The classic triad of symptoms resulting from pathologic changes associated with PIH are:

   a.

   b.

   c.

9. The major distinguishing cardinal sign between preeclampsia and eclamptic is:

10. HELLP is an acronym for the major pathologic findings of HELLP syndrome. What do the letters stand for?

    H:

    EL:

    LP:

11. Elena is a diabetic who is now in the third trimester of pregnancy. What complications could possibly develop at this time?

12. Because there are many potential fetal complications associated with diabetes in pregnancy, list four kinds of fetal monitoring that will be done.

    a.

    b.

    c.

    d.

13. Mary is a Class II cardiac patient in labor. Identify the two most common complications for which she is at risk.

    a.

    b.

14. List four nursing actions which should be implemented during Mary's labor.

    a.

    b.

    c.

    d.

UNIT IV: ADAPTATION IN THE INTRAPARTUM PERIOD

Multiple Choice Exercise of Critical Content

Circle the most correct answer.

Terri, a 17 year old primigravida, is admitted to labor and delivery during her 32nd week of pregnancy from the health care providers office because the following symptoms were present. She gained 10 pounds since her last visit a week age, her blood pressure was 168/100, she had +2 albumin in her urine. Terri said her hands and feet have been very swollen for the past four days and yesterday she developed a headache that will not go away. Admission orders include: absolute bed rest; 1200- calorie, low-salt, high-protein diet; check blood pressure, pulse, and FHT q 2 hrs; phenobarbital gr. 1/2 QID; weigh every am; urinalysis for albumin every 4 hrs; intake and output. Terri's diagnosis is preeclampsia.

1. Bed rest is essential for Terri, because it:
    a. Prevents eclampsia.
    b. Mobilizes tissue fluid, thereby lowering blood pressure.
    c. Improves circulation and decreases leg edema.
    d. Prevents premature labor and delivery.

2. The health care provider orders IV magnesium sulfate to be started on Terri. Magnesium sulfate is a:
    a. Vasodilator and anticonvulsant.
    b. Central nervous system depressant and vasopressor.
    c. Sedative and antihypertensive.
    d. Diuretic and antihypertensive.

3. You are assessing Terri while administering the magnesium sulfate and find respirations to be 12, DTRs absent, urine output for the past 4 hours of 90 ml. What would you do?
    a. Administer calcium gluconate immediately.
    b. Administer only half the dose of magnesium sulfate.
    c. Continue the magnesium sulfate as ordered.
    d. Stop the magnesium sulfate and notify the health care provider.

4. A low-salt, high-protein diet was ordered for Terri:
    a. To limit the carbohydrate intake.
    b. To prevent further weight gain.
    c. To provide a low-fat intake.
    d. Because preeclampsia is prevalent in poorly balanced low-protein diets.

5. The Phenobarbital was ordered for Terri because it acts as a:
   a. Sedative.
   b. Hypnotic.
   c. Antihypertensive.
   d. Stimulant.

6. If Terri's diagnosis had been eclampsia, she would have probably displayed which of the following symptoms?
   a. Concentrated, scant urine.
   b. Convulsion(s), with or without coma.
   c. Rise in blood pressure.
   d. All of the above symptoms.

7. Because of Terri's diagnosis, she is at increased risk for:
   a. Complete abortion.
   b. Placenta previa.
   c. Abruptio placentae.
   d. None of the above.

8. The number of diabetic women who become pregnant has:
   a. Markedly increased since the introduction of insulin.
   b. Slightly decreased since the introduction of insulin.
   c. Remained the same since the introduction of insulin.
   d. Markedly decreased since the introduction of insulin.

9. The pregnant diabetic woman is at increased risk for:
   a. Fetal macrosomia.
   b. Pregnancy induced hypertension.
   c. Fetal congenital anomalies.
   d. All of the above are correct.

10. Sonya, gravida 1, has mitral valve prolapse and has been placed on prophylactic antibiotics during labor. She asks you why she need this medicine. Your best answer would be:
    a. To prevent the chance of developing a sexually transmitted disease.
    b. To fight against toxoplasmosis because she owns a cat.
    c. To prevent development of bacterial endocarditis.
    d. To help her be allowed to push during the second stage of labor.

UNIT IV: ADAPTATION IN THE INTRAPARTUM PERIOD

True and False Exercise of Critical Content

The following statements require you to assess whether or not they are true or false. If the statement is false, rewrite it so that it is correct.

1. The use of tocolytic therapy for preterm labor has a tendency to decrease the woman's heart rate. (True/False).

2. If fetal lung immaturity is confirmed by an L/S ratio of less than 2.0, the woman may be given betamethasone. (True/False).

3. Home monitoring is cost effective in comparison to long-term hospitalization when preterm labor occurs. (True/False).

4. The greatest risk following premature ruptured membranes is intrauterine infection. (True/False).

5. The goal of care in medical complications is to provide a family-centered experience while monitoring and supporting maternal status throughout the childbearing cycle. (True/False).

Critical Thinking Exercise

1. Sherrika has been admitted with a diagnosis of preterm labor. Determine the primary nursing responsibilities in stabilizing Sherrika's problem.

2. Propose a list of nurse's responsibilities when a woman experiences an adverse reaction to beta-sympathomimetic or magnesium sulfate tocolytic therapy.

3. Donita is a type 1 diabetic that just gave birth to a 12 pound 8 ounce girl. Compare Donita's postpartum course to a nondiabetic postpartum patient.

CHAPTER 28

Nursing Care of the Family in the Postpartum Period

Overview

Mother-baby care focuses on one nurse caring for the physiologic needs of both mother and neonate, and providing emotional support and education of the new family. It is based on the acknowledgment that maternal-child health is based not only on physical dimensions, but on psychological, social, and economic dimensions as well. This chapter addresses the normal adaptations and needs of the beginning new family.

Learning Objectives

After studying the material in this chapter, the student will be able to:

- Describe the normal physiologic adaptations occurring in the postpartum period.

- Describe typical psychological adaptations occurring in the parents and family of a newborn.

- Discuss important aspects of the postpartum nursing assessment.

- Identify common nursing diagnoses presented during the postpartum period.

- Describe critical aspects of nursing care for the postpartum woman after vaginal birth and for the postpartum woman after cesarean delivery.

- Develop a nursing care plan for the postpartum woman after vaginal birth.

- Identify common paternal or partner adaptations in the postpartum period.

- Develop a nursing care plan for the postpartum woman after cesarean delivery.

- Discuss important areas of teaching to promote effective self-care and care of the infant.

UNIT V: ADAPTATION IN THE POSTPARTUM PERIOD

Application of Key Terms

Match the definitions in column two with the key terms in column one.

____ 1. Afterpains
____ 2. Boggy uterus
____ 3. Diastasis recti abdominis
____ 4. Engorgement
____ 5. Fundus
____ 6. Involution
____ 7. Let-down reflex
____ 8. Lochia
____ 9. Micturition
____ 10. Postpartum hemorrhage
____ 11. Thrombosis
____ 12. Uterine atony

A. the formation, development, or existence of a blood clot within the vascular system.

B. Hyperemia; local congestion; excessive fullness, for example, of the breast.

C. The voiding of urine.

D. Loss of 500 ml or more of blood from the uterus after completion of the third stage of labor.

E. Uterine contractions that cause pain during the first few days after childbirth.

F. Separation of the abdominal recti muscles.

G. The upper most part of the uterus between the insertions of the fallopian tubes.

H. Reduction in the size of the uterus following delivery.

I. Discharge of blood, mucus, and tissue that flows from the uterus in the postpartum period.

J. A reflex caused by increased oxytocin from the pituitary gland resulting in contractions of the breasts that force milk into the nipple ducts.

K. Lack of uterine muscle tone.

L. A soft and difficult to locate uterus.

Short Answer Exercise of Critical Content

1. Most of the physiological changes of pregnancy that are reversible return to their prepregnant state by the end of _____ weeks.

2. This six-week period is known as the _____.

3. Following delivery there is an immediate weight loss of approximately _____ pounds.

4. This immediate loss is accounted for by the weight of the _____, _____, and _____.

5. In addition to a blood loss of about _____ cc, additional fluid is lost through _____ and _____.

6. After delivery of the placenta, there is a sudden decrease in three hormones: _____, _____, and _____.

7. The fluid produced by the breast during the third trimester and in the first postpartum days is called _____.

8. Breast milk production begins around the _____ postpartum day.

9. When breasts are overdistended and painful, they are said to be _____.

NURSING CARE OF THE FAMILY IN THE POSTPARTUM PERIOD

10. The milk let-down reflex is dependent on the production of endogenous _____ which is stimulated by _____.

11. The return of the uterus to its prepregnant state is called _____.

12. The sloughing of the uterine lining is called _____.

13. The last site for the endometrium to be restored is the _____ site.

14. Intermittent uterine contractions are called _____.

15. Describe the anatomic position where you would expect to find the fundus of the involuting uterus at each of the time periods listed below.

   a. 1 to 2 hours after delivery:

   b. 12 hours after delivery:

   c. 3 days after delivery:

   d. 9 days after delivery:

Multiple Choice Exercise of Critical Content

Circle the most correct answer.

Joy is a gravida 2 para 2 who gave birth to a 7 pound 10 ounce baby boy. She had a midline episiotomy after pushing for two hours. She plans to breastfeed her infant. She has just been transferred to the mother-baby unit and part of your admission procedure is to assess Joy.

1. You palpate Joy's fundus. It should be located:
   a. At the level of the symphysis pubis.
   b. At the level of the umbilucus.
   c. Midway between the rimbilicus and symphysis pubis.
   d. Two finger breadths below the umbilicus.

2. The lochia should have a:
   a. Foul odor and be a large amount of blood.
   b. Foul odor and be dark brown with red streaks.
   c. Characteristic fleshy odor; clear colored and of moderate amount.
   d. Characteristic fleshy odor; bloody and of moderate amount.

UNIT V: ADAPTATION IN THE POSTPARTUM PERIOD

3. You inspect Joy's perineum and find it to be:
   a. Edematous, painful to pressure, and displaying a clear discharge.
   b. Edematous, painful to pressure, and perhaps displaying hemorrhoids.
   c. Intensely painful, separation of the lop edge of the episiotomy, with clear drainage.
   d. Red; clear drainage and large hemorrhoids.

4. The postpartum uterus must be carefully assessed because of the danger of postpartum hemorrhage, which is most likely to occur in a:
   a. Primipara.
   b. Multipara.
   c. Woman who has just delivered twins.
   d. Woman who delivered a low-birth-weight infant.

5. The lochia is an indicator of the rate of healing of the uterus. In which of the following sequences does it appear?
   a. Alba, rubra, serosa.
   b. Rubra, alba, serosa.
   c. Rubra, serosa, alba.
   d. Serosa, rubra, alba.

6. The next morning you begin your shift by assessing Joy again. You find that her uterus is somewhat enlarged, slightly boggy, and displaced to the right side. What would be your first nursing intervention?
   a. Administer an oxytocic drug immediately.
   b. Have Joy void, then recheck her fundus.
   c. Check the consistency of her fundus every 15 minutes.
   d. Massage the uterus vigorously and firmly until it becomes very firm.

7. You assist Joy with breastfeeding. Her breasts should be:
   a. Soft to filling and secreting colostrum.
   b. Engorged and secreting colostrum.
   c. Soft and secreting milk.
   d. Engorged and not secreting any fluid.

8. You observe Joy as she breastfeeds her infant. Clues to the nature of attachment behaviors would include:
   a. Presence and duration of eye contact.
   b. Comments that the infant looks like her husband.
   c. She uses a soft voice and rocking motion to soothe the infant.
   d. All of the above are positive clues of attachment.

9. Darnita has chosen to bottle feed her infant. She is three days postdelivery and her breasts have become engorged. Which of the following steps may be helpful to the non-nursing mother?

    a. Do not stimulate the breast.

    b. Apply ice packs to the breast.

    c. Support the breasts with a snugly fitting bra.

    d. All of the above may be helpful.

10. The most common cause of sore nipples is:

    a. Allowing the nipples to air dry after feedings.

    b. Using a nipple shield to get the baby started.

    c. Improper positioning of the neonate on the nipple.

    d. Application of vitamin E, aloe vera, or lanolin.

True and False Exercise of Critical Content

The following statements require you to assess whether or not they are true of false. If the statement is false, rewrite it so that it is correct.

1. Bowel function is usually reestablished by the end of the first postpartum week as the woman's mobility, appetite, and fluid intake increase. (True/False).

2. Most of the changes that occur during pregnancy and the intrapartum period are reversed by the second to fourth week after delivery. (True/False).

3. Parental adaptation in the postpartum period involves taking on new role responsibilities and behaviors, readjusting relationships with significant others, and beginning an acquaintance with the long-awaited newborn. (True/False).

4. Many young children may respond negatively to the birth of a sibling; they may demonstrate some degree of regression, heightened dependency needs, and aggression directed at the newborn. (True/False).

5. Men experience profound physiologic changes but do not have similar needs to integrate the birth into their life experience. (True/False).

6. The nurse should encourage the father or partner to hold and care for the newborn, while acknowledging the concerns and insecurity most new fathers feel. (True/False).

Critical Thinking Exercise

1. Summarize significant deviations in maternal vital signs that would indicate complications in the postpartum recovery process.

2. Belinda delivered yesterday and today is complaining of pain in her left leg. She has a positive Homen's sign and edema in her left leg. Prepare Belinda for treatment of deep vein thrombosis. Formulate a plan of care for Belinda.

3. Compare and contrast postpartum care of a normal vaginal delivery patient and a cesarean delivery patient.

CHAPTER 29

Postpartum Complications

Overview

The postpartum period is a time of profound physical and psychological adaptation. When problems develop during this time, they can become overwhelming. Serious postpartum medical problems have an impact on individual coping as well as on early family formation, breastfeeding, and the woman's future health status. This chapter discusses the most common and most life-threatening postpartum complications.

Learning Objectives

After studying the material in this chapter, the student will be able to:

- Identify the most common complications that occur during the postpartum period.

- Describe predisposing factors for infections of the reproductive and urinary tracts and modes of entry and diffusion of infections.

- Discuss common causes of early and late postpartum hemorrhage.

- Explain treatment modalities and common procedures used in the management of postpartum complications.

- Discuss psychological and social problems encountered in postpartum women experiencing complications.

- Identify the goals of nursing care, appropriate nursing interventions, and their rationale for women with specific postpartum problems.

UNIT V: ADAPTATION IN THE POSTPARTUM PERIOD

Application of Key Terms

Match the definitions in column two with the key terms in column one.

_____ 1. Bacteriuria
_____ 2. Curettage
_____ 3. Cystitis
_____ 4. Embolus
_____ 5. Endometritis
_____ 6. Hematuria
_____ 7. Mastitis
_____ 8. Oliguria
_____ 9. Parametritis
_____ 10. Peritonitis
_____ 11. Placenta accreta
_____ 12. Placenta increta
_____ 13. Placenta percreta
_____ 14. Postpartum infection

A. Blood in the urine.
B. Inflammation of the parametrium.
C. Presence of bacteria in the urine.
D. Infection of the urinary bladder.
E. Diminished production of urine.
F. Inflammation of the peritoneum.
G. Acute inflammation of the breast caused by bacteria entering a cracked nipple during lactation.
H. Clot or other plug carried by a blood vessel and blocking a smaller one.
I. Inflammation of the endometrium.
J. Scraping of the inner surface of the uterus with a curet to remove its lining or content.
K. Placenta in which the cotyledons have invaded the uterine musculature.
L. Type of placenta accreta in which the myometrium is invaded to the serosa of the peritoneum covering the uterus.
M. Postpartum sepsis; a major cause of maternal morbidity and mortality.
N. Form of placenta accreta in which the chorionic villi invade the myometrium.

Short Answer Exercise of Critical Content

1. List five predisposing factors in uterine atony.

   a.

   b.

   c.

   d.

   e.

POSTPARTUM COMPLICATIONS

2. Summarize the classifications of perineal and vaginal lacerations.

   a. First degree:

   b. Second degree

   c. Third degree:

   d. Fourth degree:

3. Uterine inversion is a rare but dramatic postpartum complication. List three causes of uterine inversion.

   a.

   b.

   c.

4. List five important nursing interventions to prevent postpartum infection.

   a.

   b.

   c.

   d.

   e.

5. It is important to assess every postpartum patient for signs and symptoms of superficial or deep vein thrombosis. Signs and symptoms of SVT or DVT include:

   a.

   b.

   c.

   d.

   e.

Multiple Choice Exercise of Critical Content

Circle the most correct answer.

1. Regina, gravida 4, para 4, delivered a healthy 9 pound 10 ounce boy following a lengthy labor. She was delivered vaginally by use of the Mity Vac. This is Regina's second postpartum day and during your assessment, Regina complains that she is having a lot of perineal pain, has problems sitting, and feels very swollen in her bottom. You suspect and examine her for:

   a. Cystitis
   b. Postpartum hemorrhage
   c. Postpartum infection
   d. Vulvar hematoma

2. Deirdre gave birth to a 7 pound 14 ounce girl a week ago. She telephones you to ask your advice. She has begun having lochia rubra again for the past two days and is using nine to ten maternity pads a day. You would suspect which of the following?

   a. Endometritis
   b. Subinvolution
   c. Menstruation
   d. Parametritis

3. The clinical manifestations of a localized episiotomy infection would probably include:

   a. Complaint of severe discomfort and oral temperature of 99.6°F.
   b. Reddened, edematous tissue with foul odor.
   c. Reddened, edematous and bruised tissue.
   d. Approximated skin edges with some edematous tissue.

POSTPARTUM COMPLICATIONS

4. During your assessment of Shana, 2 days postpartum, you discover a positive Homen's sign. A positive Homen's sign is elicited when:

    a. The patient stands and pain is felt in her foot.

    b. The foot is dorsiflexed while the knee is held flat and pain is felt in the leg.

    c. The knee is flexed, the foot is extended, and pain is felt in her leg.

    d. The knee is held flat, the foot is rotated, and pain is felt in her leg.

5. Shana was diagnosed with thrombophlebitis and is receiving heparin therapy. You need to watch Shana closely for signs of heparin overdose which include:

    a. Dysuria.

    b. Epistaxis, hematuria, and dysuria.

    c. Hematuria, ecchymosis, and epistaxis.

    d. Hematuria, ecchymosis, and vertigo.

6. The next morning you are assessing Shana and she suddenly complains of dyspnea and chest pain. Shana has most likely developed:

    a. A drug reaction to heparin.

    b. An inflammatory reaction.

    c. Another thrombophlebitis.

    d. Pulmonary embolism.

7. Juanita suffered a prolapsed uterus and after several attempts the health care provider was unable to replace the uterus. Juanita needs to be prepared for:

    a. Continual manual replacement attempts.

    b. Immediate emergency hysterectomy.

    c. Administration of uterine tonics.

    d. Dilatation and curettage.

8. Kim had an infection in her episiotomy one week after delivery. When she comes in for her six-week check-up she complains of temperature spikes to 105°F; nausea, vomiting, and diarrhea; and acute abdominal pain. The health care provider diagnoses:

    a. Mastitis.

    b. Endometritis.

    c. Peritonitis.

    d. Cystitis.

9. Shelby is breastfeeding her newborn and has developed mastitis. The clinical signs and symptoms of mastitis include:

   a. A hard, warm nodular area in the outer quadrant of the breast.

   b. Cessation of lactation with bloody discharge.

   c. Marked engorgement and excessive pain.

   d. Marked engorgement, high temperature, chills, and pain.

10. Julie is in the "New Beginning" program. When the nurse makes the home visit on the fifth postpartum day, she finds Julie tearful, socially withdrawn, and despondent. Julie is most likely experiencing:

    a. The first signs of infection.

    b. Adaptation and bonding reactions.

    c. Postpartum blues or depression.

    d. Signs of thromboembolic disease.

Matching Exercise of Critical Content

Match the following postpartum complication for which the woman is at greatest risk with the following situations.

	Situations	Complication
___	1. Kay, gravida 5, para 5; labor lasted 2 hours; baby weighted 9 pounds 12 ounces.	A. Postpartum hemorrhage
___	2. Donna, gravida 1, para 1; age 36; pre-pregnancy history of essential hypertension.	B. Postpartum infection
___	3. Veronica, gravida 2; para 2; labor induced after PROM 24 hours duration.	C. Postpartum eclampsia
___	4. Shawntrice, gravida 3, para 3; previous history of suicidal tendency; husband absent because of occupation.	D. Postpartum psychosis/mood disorder/blues

True and False Exercise of Critical Content

The following statements require you to assess whether or not they are true or false. If the statement is false, rewrite it so that it is correct.

1. Cesarean birth does not increase the risk of maternal mortality or morbidity. (True/False).

2. The most important indicators of potential postpartum hemorrhage are pulse and blood pressure. (True/False).

POSTPARTUM COMPLICATIONS

3. Preeclampsia may contribute to postpartum hemorrhage by altering the platelet count. (True/False).

4. Adele experienced an abruptio placenta. She is not at increased risk for postpartum hemorrhage. (True/False).

5. Marilee has symptoms of postpartum infection. Before administering the first dose of antibiotic, the nurse should establish that Marilee is not allergic to the drug. (True/False).

6. Scant lochia on the third postpartum day is a potential indicator of infection. (True/False).

7. Dinah's postpartum assessment findings include costovertebral angle tenderness. This is a sign of cystitis. (True/False).

8. Thrombophlebitis is a complication caused by the hormone balance of pregnancy. (True/False).

Critical Thinking Exercise

1. Meredith suffered a postpartum hemorrhage and consequently hypovolemia and shock. Explain the signs of hypovolemia and compensated shock in the postpartum woman. Determine primary nursing responsibilities when shock is identified.

2. Explain to a group of postpartum mothers activities they can perform to reduce the recurrence of a urinary tract infection.

3. When you walk into Lori's postpartum room you find her crying for no apparent reason. Differentiate between postpartum blues and postpartum affective mood disorder (depression).

4. Propose strategies that the nurse can use to effectively assess the postpartum mood or emotional status.

CHAPTER 30

Assessment of the Neonate

Overview

Major physiologic and behavioral adaptations must be made before the neonatal period is safely concluded at the 28th day of life. The extrauterine adjustments made during the first 24 hours are particularly critical to the neonate's chances for survival. This chapter discusses the major physiologic and behavioral adaptations the neonate must undergo after birth.

Learning Objectives

After studying the material in this chapter, the student will be able to:

- Describe the major physiologic adaptations required of the neonate in the first 24 hours of life.

- Describe the major behavioral adaptations required of the neonate in the first 24 hours of life.

- Outline essential steps in the process of newborn assessment.

- Describe normal physical and behavioral findings in the newborn.

- Explain the purpose of a gestational age assessment and describe the components of this assessment.

Application of Key Terms

Match the definitions in column two with the key terms in column one.

1. Acrocyanosis
2. Caput succedaneum
3. Cephalhematoma
4. Erythema toxicum
5. Frenulum linguae
6. Full-term infant
7. Habituation
8. Hypoglycemia
9. Icterus neonatorum
10. Infant
11. Jaundice
12. Meconium
13. Milia
14. Molding
15. Mongolian spots
16. Moro reflex
17. Neonate
18. Nonshivering thermogenesis
19. Plethora
20. Polycythemia
21. Pseudomenstruation
22. Reactivity
23. Rugae
24. Vernix caseosa
25. Webbing

A. Graywhite, cheeselike sebaceous material that covers the skin of the fetus to protect it from the amniotic fluid.

B. Infant from birth through the first 28 days of life.

C. Normal process by which the fetal head is shaped during labor as it passes through the tight birth canal.

D. Child under 1 year of age.

E. Fecal material discharged by the newborn, green black in color and consisting of mucus, bile, and epithelial shreds.

F. Cyanosis of the extremities in most infants at birth; may persist for 7 to 10 days.

G. Fold of mucous membrane extending from the floor of the mouth to the inferior portion of the tongue and restraining its movement.

H. Physiologic jaundice in the newborn.

I. Excessive number of red blood cells.

J. Defensive reflex present from birth to 3 months of age that causes the infant to draw its arms across the chest in an embracing manner when startled.

K. Swelling produced on the fetal head during labor

L. Yellow discoloration of the skin, whites of the eyes, mucous membranes, and body fluids caused by excessive bilirubin in the blood.

M. Localized collection of blood beneath the periosteum of the newborn skull caused by disruption of blood vessels during birth.

N. Minute white cysts on the skin of newborns caused by obstruction of hair follicles.

O. Infant born between 38 and 42 weeks of gestation.

P. Benign bluish pigmentation over the lower back and buttocks that may be present at birth, especially in dark-skinned races.

Q. The primary method of heat production in neonates.

R. Three distinct stages, which begin at birth, are characterized by waking and sleep states and by rapid changes in physiologic functioning.

S. A deep red coloration of the skin, often exaggerated with crying.

T. A benign maculopapular rash with an erythematous base and a pale yellow papule.

U. Folds or creases in the skin especially in the scrotum.

V. Presence of a membrane between fingers or toes.

W. Mucoid vaginal discharge, which may be blood-tinged.

X. The ability of the newborn to diminish a response to specific repeated stimuli.

Y. A blood glucose level of less than 30 mg/dL during the first 72 hours of life.

UNIT V: ADAPTATION IN THE POSTPARTUM PERIOD

Short Answer Exercise of Critical Content

1. Fetal lungs must be developed sufficiently to produce _____.

2. Four major categories of respiratory stimuli have been identified. List the categories and briefly describe each.

    a.

    b.

    c.

    d.

3. With clamping of the umbilical cord and initiation of the first breath, dramatic changes occur in the cardiovascular system of the neonate. List those three changes.

    a.

    b.

    c.

4. Thermoregulation is a critical aspect of the newborn's transition to extrauterine life. Explain what happens if a newborn does not stay warm.

5. The _____ coagulation factors and a prolonged blood coagulation time in the neonate are deficient at birth because the intestinal tract does not harbor bacteria that manufacture _____.

6. The newborn's gastric capacity is limited in the first day of life to approximately _____ to _____ mL and increases to _____ mL by 3 to 4 days of age.

7. Most infants void within _____ from birth. Uric acid crystals excreted in the urine leave _____ stains in the diaper. The baby may void as many as _____ times a day.

8. The newborn's iron reserve lasts until approximately the _____ month of life.

9. The newborn's neurologic system is _____.

ASSESSMENT OF THE NEONATE

10. Newborns experience predictable behavior patterns following birth. Describe each of the reactive periods; list the major behavioral characteristics of each; and suggest nursing care required during the stage.

    a. First period of reactivity

    Behavior characteristics:

    Nursing care:

    b. Period of inactivity

    Behavioral characteristics:

    Nursing care:

    c. Second period of reactivity

    Behavioral characteristics:

    Nursing care:

Multiple Choice Exercise of Critical Content

Circle the most correct answer.

1. Christie delivers a 7 pound 12 ounce boy that is 21 inches long. Bill, the proud new father, wants to know if this is a normal size. You response would be that the baby is:

    a. Above average weight and above the average length.

    b. Below the average weight and below the average length.

    c. The average weight and above the average length.

    d. The average weight and the average length.

2. Part of your assessment includes observing the newborn's breathing pattern. A full-term newborn's breathing pattern is predominantly:

    a. Abdominal with synchronous chest movements.

    b. Chest breathing with nasal flaring.

    c. Diaphragmatic with chest lag.

    d. Shallow with irregular respirations.

3. You also take an apical pulse. The average expected apical pulse range of a full-term, quiet, awake newborn would be:

   a. 80-100 beats per minute.
   b. 100-120 beats per minute.
   c. 120-140 beats per minute.
   d. 150-180 beats per minute.

4. The newborn received an injection of vitamin K because:

   a. The newborn's liver does not produce enough vitamin K to handle neonatal coagulation problems.
   b. Hemolysis of the fetal red blood cells increases coagulation requirements.
   c. Newborns are susceptible to avitaminosis.
   d. Newborns lack intestinal bacteria with which to synthesize vitamin K.

5. The newborn's eyes were treated with Ilotycin ophthalmic ointment. The nurse explains to Christie and Bill that the purpose of this treatment is to:

   a. Destroy an infectious exudate caused by staphylococcus.
   b. Destroy gonococcal organisms, potentially acquired from the birth canal.
   c. Prevent potentially harmful exudate from invading the tear ducts.
   d. Prevent the eyelids from sticking together.

6. Bill states that the newborn must be cold because his hands and feet are blue. You explain that this is a common and temporary condition called:

   a. Acrocyanosis.
   b. Erythema neonatorum.
   c. Harlequin color.
   d. Vernix caseosa

7. The nurse should explain to Christie and Bill what to expect of their baby. Which of the following symptoms are normal in a newborn infant?

   a. Hiccoughing and sneezing.
   b. Slight jaundice that may appear on day three.
   c. Movements due to startling the infant when the crib is jarred.
   d. All of the above are normal in a newborn.

ASSESSMENT OF THE NEONATE

8. Sheela, an African-American, wonders who spanked her newborn girl and left bruises across her buttocks. You explain to Sheela that these are a temporary condition called:

   a. Vanugo.

   b. Vascular nevi.

   c. Mongolian spots.

   d. Nevus flammeus.

9. When examining Sheela's newborn, you note uneven skin folds of the buttocks and a click when doing Ortolani's test. You know this is a sign that the baby probably has:

   a. Polydactyly.

   b. Hip dysplasia.

   c. Clubfoot.

   d. Webbing.

10. When you use the Ballard scale to estimate the gestational age of Susheela's baby, you find thick and leathery skin with deep cracking and significant peeling. This is considered a sign of:

    a. A premature infant.

    b. A mature infant.

    c. A postmature infant.

    d. A large-for-gestational-age infant.

Matching Exercise of Critical Content

Match the following findings with either:

_____ 1. Appears at birth.

_____ 2. Does not increase in size.

_____ 3. Never crosses suture lines.

_____ 4. Crosses suture lines.

_____ 5. Increases in size for 2-3 days.

_____ 6. Appears several hours after birth.

_____ 7. Localized sof-tissue edema.

_____ 8. Complications include: jaundice, skull fracture, intracranial bleeding.

A. Caput Succedaneum

B. Cephalhematoma

UNIT V: ADAPTATION IN THE POSTPARTUM PERIOD

True and False Exercise of Critical Content

The following statements require you to assess whether or not they are true or false. If the statement is false, rewrite it so that it is correct.

1. Respirations in the neonate are triggered by increased PaO_2, decreased $PaCO_2$ and decreased pH. (True/False).

2. Hyperbilirubinemia develops when elevated levels of glucuronyl transferase metabolize fetal RBC s. (True/False).

3. Glycogenolysis releases glucose into the neonate's bloodstream, maintaining a blood glucose level of 90 mg/ml. (True/False).

4. The neonate's bowel is sterile, causing a deficiency in Vitamin K and a potential for bleeding disorders. (True/False).

5. Nonshivering thermogenesis and increased metabolism are the newborn's methods of heat production. (True/False).

6. At birth, the newborn has elevated levels of each of the immunoglobulins IgA, IgE, IgG, and IgM, providing protection against infections. (True/False).

ASSESSMENT OF THE NEONATE

Critical Thinking Exercise

1. Compare and contrast the types of jaundice in a newborn; physiologic; pathologic; true breast milk jaundice; and jaundice associated with breastfeeding.

2. You are performing a newborn assessment on Trina's newborn. Explain to Trina the significance of the gestational age assessment.

3. It has been two hours since Melissa gave birth to a seven pound baby boy. She is very frustrated with trying to breastfeed her newborn son. All he seems to want to do is sleep. Determine how sleep-wake states influence parent-newborn interactions. Organize a plan to assist Melissa with breastfeeding.

CHAPTER 31

Nursing Care of the Low-Risk Neonate

Overview

The nurse can make the neonate's adjustment to extrauterine life less traumatic by adapting the environment, providing individualized nursing care, and facilitating the parent-newborn attachment process. This chapter deals with nursing care designed to support physiologic and behavioral adaptation and to facilitate the parent-newborn attachment process during ongoing care in a variety of settings.

Learning Objectives

After studying the material in this chapter, the student will be able to:

- Discuss how hospital environments influence neonatal adaptation.
- Describe specific nursing interventions that facilitate stabilization of physiologic functions in the transitional period.
- Describe specific nursing interventions that promote the parent-newborn interaction.
- Discuss common nursing interventions used to prevent potential neonatal complications.
- Formulate a nursing care plan for daily care of the neonate.
- Develop an appropriate parent-teaching discharge plan.
- Describe newborn screening tests and discuss their importance in preparation for discharge.
- Discuss the risks and benefits of circumcision.

Application of Key Terms

Match the definitions in column two with the key terms in column one.

_____ 1. Aspiration
_____ 2. Attachment
_____ 3. Circumcision
_____ 4. Cradle cap
_____ 5. Demand feeding
_____ 6. Diurnal rhythm
_____ 7. Hyperbilirubinemia
_____ 8. Hypoglycemia
_____ 9. Hypothermia
_____ 10. Omphalitis
_____ 11. Ophthalmia neonatorum
_____ 12. Polycythemia
_____ 13. Prophylaxis
_____ 14. Regurgitation
_____ 15. Rooming-in

A. Excessive concentration of bilirubin in the blood that may lead to jaundice.
B. Infection of the umbilicus.
C. Excessive number of red blood cells.
D. Inhaling mucus, meconium, or stomach contents into the lungs that may result in atelectasis or pneumonia.
E. Removal of all or part of the prepuce, or the foreskin, in the male infant.
F. Practice of allowing the infant to determine the frequency of feedings and amount of milk ingested.
G. Protection from or prevention of a disease or event.
H. Affiliative tie formed after a period of mutual stimulation and response.
I. Seborrheic dermatitis of the newborn that appears on the head, scalp, and face of the newborn.
J. Purulent conjunctivitis of the newborn.
K. A blood glucose level of less than 30 mg/dL during the first 72 hours of life.
L. An arrangement that allows mothers the opportunity to keep their newborns with them in the postpartum unit.
M. Having a body temperature below normal.
N. A backward flowing of fluids to the mouth from the stomach.
O. Patterns of physiologic functioning occurring with predictable frequency on a daily basis.

Short Answer Exercise of Critical Content

1. A hematocrit above _____ to _____ % may be indicative of polycythemia.
2. When providing direct care to an infant, rings and watches should be removed because they are common _____.
3. A blood glucose level less than _____ mg/dl during the first 72 hours of life in the full term neonate is considered hypoglycemic.
4. Seizures and apnea are potential complications of untreated _____.
5. When inspecting a neonate who may be suffering from hyperbilirubinemia, the _____ or _____ should be inspected first.
6. The initiation of early and frequent feedings can help to reduce serum _____ levels.
7. _____ stress can increase the risk of hypoglycemia.

UNIT V: ADAPTATION IN THE POSTPARTUM PERIOD

8. Propose the rationale for providing the infant with a first feeding of sterile water.

9. Explain the differences between a circumcision performed with a Yellen clamp and one performed with a Plastibell.

10. Prepare answers to the following parental questions at the time of discharge of their infant.

    a. How warm does the room have to be when I bathe my baby?

    b. Should my baby's foreskin be retracted during his bath?

    c. Can I put the baby in a small tub to bathe him the day he goes home?

    d. Is it really necessary to put the baby in an infant car seat to take him home?

    e. How will I know if my baby is getting sick?

Multiple Choice Exercise of Critical Content

Circle the most correct answer

1. Which of the following statements regarding psychological growth of the newborn infant are correct?
    a. The infant's need for contact with a mother figure is greater that the need for food.
    b. The infant perceives the outside world as the source of gratification of basic needs.
    c. The cry is the infant's only defense mechanism.
    d. All the above are correct statements regarding psychological growth of the newborn.

2. Regina is concerned because her baby weighs less on day 2 than she did when she was born. You explain that normal neonatal weight loss after birth:
    a. Can be prevented with adequate nutritional intake.
    b. Can range from 5 to 10% in healthy babies.
    c. Occurs only in very large or premature babies.
    d. Reflects a potentially harmful fluid imbalance.

NURSING CARE OF THE LOW-RISK NEONATE

3. Regina is rooming-in. Which of the following statements is true about rooming-in.
   a. All mothers should have their babies at their bedsides so that they may learn the techniques of infant care.
   b. The rooming-in plan reduces the total number of professional personnel needed.
   c. The rooming-in plan should be flexible so that if a mother does not wish her baby at her bedside the baby may return to the nursery.
   d. A baby who has been at the mother's bedside should never be returned to the nursery because of the danger of infecting other babies.

4. Regina is inspecting her baby and asks you why the cord and part of the abdomen is purple. You reply:
   a. Alcohol turns the cord purple.
   b. The cord was painted with Triple dye after birth.
   c. The cord is infected, that is why it is purple.
   d. The soap the baby was bathed with after birth turned the cord purple.

5. Alberta's baby boy was circumcised early this morning. You tell Alberta that she and the baby can be discharged home after:
   a. All bleeding stops.
   b. The penis is healed.
   c. The blood work results come from the lab.
   d. The infant voids.

Matching Exercise of Critical Content

Match the following with the appropriate defining characteristic.

Terms	Defining Characteristic
1. Football hold	A. Prevents bleeding
2. 25% of the infant's total body length	B. Single most important anti-infection measure.
	C. Baby's head is supported by adult's hand.
3. Handwashing	D. Head.
4. Vitamin K	E. Increased risk of hypoglycemia.
5. PKU	F. A screening test.
6. Cold stress	

True and False Exercise of Critical Content

The following statements require you to assess whether or not they are true or false. If the statement is false, rewrite it so that it is correct.

1. Rooming-in means that labor, delivery, and care of the infant following delivery all occur in the same room. (True/False).

2. Family centered nursing care promotes the neonate's adjustment to extrauterine life. (True/False).

3. The problem of ineffective thermoregulation generally is not seen in the transitional period. (True/False).

4. Infants demonstrate a wide variation in elimination patterns in the first few days of life. (True/False).

5. There is no need to include signs and symptoms of illness in a parent teaching discharge plan if the parents already have children at home. (True/False).

6. A PKU should be obtained only after the infant has had 2-3 days of milk or formula. (True/False).

7. Circumcisions are associated with sleep pattern disturbances. (True/False).

8. There is no need to limit family members that visit the nursery as long as they wear cover gowns. (True/False).

NURSING CARE OF THE LOW-RISK NEONATE

Critical Thinking Exercise

1. Maureen and Steve are undecided about having their baby boy circumcised. Critique the pros and cons of this procedure.

2. Develop a discharge teaching packet that parents may take home with them when the infant is discharged. Include pictures that depict procedures and develop a list of signs and symptoms of illness. Select references that include parent support/special interest groups to include.

3. Jacquelyn is unsure of what birth setting she would like to use for delivery. Compare and contrast three family centered childbirth settings with the traditional setting.

CHAPTER 32

Assessment of the At-Risk Neonate

Overview

Modern technology makes it possible to save neonates who would have died in the past. Neonatal nursing had become a specialty and nurses have advanced theoretical preparations and clinical training to function in this specialized role. This chapter defines the concept of risk assessment in the neonatal period and demonstrates how nursing assessment can be used systematically in the early recognition and treatment of potential or actual problems.

LEARNING OBJECTIVES

After studying the material in this chapter, the student will be able to:

- Identify major goals and objectives in the assessment of neonatal risk factors.

- Demonstrate the use of the Apgar score to assess the neonate's need for resuscitation after birth.

- Describe the use of umbilical cord blood pH and gas analysis in medical treatment and nursing care of the neonate.

- Demonstrate the prescribed steps in resuscitation of the neonate.

- Describe danger signals or signs in the neonate that indicate actual or potential problems.

- List signs of behavioral disorganization in the high-risk neonate.

- Describe the phases in recovery of behavioral capacities in the sick or injured neonate.

ASSESSMENT OF THE AT-RISK NEONATE

Applications of Key Terms

Match the definitions in column two with the key terms in column one.

_____ 1. Apnea
_____ 2. Asphyxia
_____ 3. Cyanosis
_____ 4. Decerebrate posture
_____ 5. Decorticate posture
_____ 6. Hypoxemia
_____ 7. Hypoxia
_____ 8. Intrauterine growth retardation
_____ 9. Low-birth-weight neonate.
_____ 10. Morbidity
_____ 11. Mortality
_____ 12. Neonatology
_____ 13. Perinatal
_____ 14. Postterm neonate
_____ 15. Preterm neonate
_____ 16. Resuscitation
_____ 17. Small-for-gestational age

A. Reduction to below physiologic levels in the supply of oxygen to tissue.
B. Pertaining to the fetal death rate.
C. Period from the 28th week of gestation through the 28th day of life.
D. Infant of any weight who falls below the tenth percentile on the intrauterine growth curve.
E. Cessation of respirations.
F. Deficiency of oxygen in the blood.
G. The condition of being diseased or sick; pertaining to the sickness rate.
H. Art and science of diagnosis and treatment of disorders of the neonate.
I. Infant born after the onset of the 42nd week of gestation.
J. Infant weighing 2500 g or less at birth, regardless of gestational age.
K. Condition caused by a lack of oxygen in the blood.
L. Fetal condition characterized by failure to grow at the expected rate.
M. A dark bluish or purplish coloration of the skin and mucous membranes due to deficient oxygenation of the blood.
N. Restoration of life after apparent death.
O. The extremities are stiff and extended, and the head is retracted.
P. Infant born before the end of the 37th week of gestation.
Q. The posture is one in which the patient is rigidly still with arms flexed, fists clenched, and the legs extended.

Short Answer Exercise of Critical Content

1. List the classic signs of respiratory distress.

2. List the major danger signs associated with the gastrointestinal system of the neonate that may be useful in identifying an infant at risk.

3. Compare and contrast the signs and symptoms of hypoglycemia, hypocalcemia, and CNS irritability in the neonate.

4. Evaluate the significance of the differences in Apgar scores.

   a. Neonates with Apgar scores of 8 to 10.

   b. Neonates with Apgar scores of 5 to 7.

   c. Neonates with Apgar scores of 3 to 4.

   d. Neonates with Apgar scores of 0 to 2.

5. List classic signs of central nervous system anomalies.

Multiple Choice Exercise of Critical Content

Circle the most correct answer.

1. Lasandra is progressing in labor when deep early decelerations are noted on the fetal monitor. When the baby is born, he has a tight nucal cord twice around his neck. The baby requires hand ventilation to initiate respirations. The baby needs to be watched closely for further signs of:

   a. Reaction to formula feeding.
   b. Exposure to too many visitors.
   c. Respiratory distress.
   d. Over heating.

2. Lasandra's baby remains cyanotic and he is moved to the special care nursery where IV fluids are started via an umbilical vein. As the nurse observes the baby, he is seen to repetitively stick his tongue out and have bicycling motions of his legs. The nurse suspects:

   a. Subtle seizures.
   b. Tonic seizures.
   c. Multifocal clonic seizures.
   d. Focal clonic seizures.

ASSESSMENT OF THE AT-RISK NEONATE

3. The baby is placed under oxygen support. You would position the baby in a neutral or sniffing position. This position.

   a. Provides an adequate flow of oxygen.

   b. Permits maximal entry of air into the lungs.

   c. Provides the infant with maximum concentration of oxygen.

   d. Permits the infant time to decompensate from the oxygen.

4. The baby remains in the special care nursery for observations. When he cries, the nurse observes a pale, gray subtle color change with increasing circumoral cyanosis. She would suspect:

   a. Transient tachypnea of the newborn.

   b. Downs syndrome.

   c. Cardiac problems or tracheoesophageal fistula.

   d. Behavioral disorders.

5. Lasandra is anxious when she visits the special care nursery because of all the equipment. The nurses best response to facilitate parent-infant interaction would be to:

   a. Assure Lasandra that she is fortunate to have the baby in a special-care nursery.

   b. Explain the equipment in simple terms; have Lasandra wash her hands; and encourage physical contact.

   c. Explain the equipment and discuss the baby's viability and continued support measures.

   d. Tell Lasandra not to worry and place a chair next to the warmer so she can observe the baby.

Matching Exercise of Critical Content

Match the following characteristics with the conditions that would be observed.

Condition	Characteristic
_____ 1. Meconium aspiration	A. Failure to produce urine in first 48 hours of life.
_____ 2. Heartbeat absent or below 60 bpm	B. Incomplete closure of fetal circulatory bypasses.
_____ 3. Bulging fontanelles	
_____ 4. Heart murmur	C. Increased intracranial pressure.
_____ 5. Obstruction to urinary flow	D. External cardiac massage.
_____ 6. Hypoglycemia	E. Deep suctioning is required.
	F. Glucose level less than 30 mg/dL.

True and False Exercise of Critical Content

The following statements require you to assess whether or not they are true or false. If the statement is false, rewrite it so that it is correct.

1. Approximately 60% of neonates requiring special care and treatment at birth can be identified through careful evaluation of the mother's prenatal history. (True/False).

2. Planning and implementation of care begins prior to the nurse identifying all significant prenatal risk factors. (True/False).

3. A 5-minute Apgar score reflects the neonate's changing condition and the adequacy of resuscitative efforts. (True/False).

4. All nurses who participate in the birth and immediate assessment of the neonate must be skilled in the basics of resuscitation developed by the AHA and AAP. (True/False).

5. The nurse should concentrate all assessments upon the newborn and ignore the parents. (True/False).

ASSESSMENT OF THE AT-RISK NEONATE

Critical Thinking Exercise

1. In the clinical setting, select a client with a high-risk infant. Analyze her understanding of the infants condition and treatments. Develop a teaching plan to meet her needs. Implement the teaching plan. Critique your experience in post- conference.

2. Carlethia has delivered a female that suffered head trauma and as result has experienced tonic seizures. Explain causes of head trauma. Recommend measures to prevent head trauma.

3. While observing deliveries, practice assigning Apgar scores to the neonate at one and five minutes post-delivery. Compare your results with those recorded on the chart. Evaluate discrepancies with your instructor or the staff.

CHAPTER 33

Nursing Care of the High-Risk Neonate

Overview

The nurse must possess the basic skills and knowledge required to recognize major neonatal complications, initiate resuscitation, and assist in stabilizing the neonate's condition. The outcome of the neonate's condition is influenced by the care received immediately after birth. This chapter describes how the nursing process can be used to accomplish the goals of nursing care in a rational and systematic manner.

Learning Objectives

After studying the material in this chapter, the student will be able to:

- Describe the implications of perinatal regionalization for families and health care provider.
- Identify nursing interventions in the care of the neonate with altered respiratory function.
- Demonstrate nursing interventions when providing neonatal nutritional needs.
- Identify principles of infection control in the special care nursery.
- Discuss nursing actions in support of parents of the high-risk neonate.
- Describe therapeutic interventions used in the prevention of hyperbilirubinemia and kernicterus.
- Identify predisposing factors in birth asphyxia.
- Explain problems of the neonate with complications related to gestational age.
- Describe care of the neonate with effects of maternal substance abuse.
- Discuss prevention of neonatal infection.
- Describe birth trauma and its results.

NURSING CARE OF THE HIGH-RISK NEONATE

Application of Key Terms

Match the definitions in column two with the key terms in column one.

1. Apnea
2. Asphyxia
3. Intrauterine growth retardation
4. Large-for-gestational age neonate
5. Low-birth-weight neonate
6. Neonatal abstinence Syndrome
7. Postterm neonate
8. Preterm neonate
9. Respiratory distress syndrome
10. Sepsis
11. Small-for-gestational age neonate

A. Infant of any weight who falls below the tenth percentile on the intrauterine growth curve.
B. Presence of pathogenic microorganisms of their toxins in blood or other tissues.
C. Disease of the newborn who is delivered before full lung maturity has occurred.
D. Infant born before the end of the 37th week of gestation.
E. Infant born after the onset of the 42nd week of gestation.
F. Infant weighing 2,500 g or less at birth, regardless of gestational age.
G. Infant of any weight who falls above the 90th percentile on the intrauterine growth curve.
H. Fetal condition characterized by failure to grow at the expected rate.
I. Condition caused by a lack of oxygen in the blood.
J. Cessation of respirations.
K. Narcotic withdrawal after birth.

Short Answer Exercise of Critical Content

1. Nursing interventions for the high-risk neonate are similar to those for the normal neonate with the possibility of increased complications. Identify four essential interventions in the care of all newborns.

    a.

    b.

    c.

    d.

UNIT V: ADAPTATION IN THE POSTPARTUM PERIOD

2. The nurse caring for the infant with a central venous line must be alert to common complications. List three complications and the relevant nursing actions for prevention/early detection of complications.

   a.

   b.

   c.

3. Identify four major complications associated with umbilical artery catheterization.

4. List three of seven potential nursing interventions related to the administration of total parenteral nutrition.

   a.

   b.

   c.

5. Describe four effects of cold stress on the neonate.

   a.

   b.

   c.

   d.

6. List four factors that are associated with the development of retrolental fibroplasia.

    a.

    b.

    c.

    d.

7. Identify at least three etiologic factors that can lead to asphyxia of the infant at birth.

    a.

    b.

    c.

8. Evidence of chronic intrauterine infection at birth might include:

    a.

    b.

    c.

9. Identify the components of a "sepsis work-up".

10. The infant suspected of, or diagnosed as having, a skull fracture is assessed closely for evidence of increased intracranial pressure secondary to hemorrhage or brain edema. Such evidence includes:

UNIT V: ADAPTATION IN THE POSTPARTUM PERIOD

Multiple Choice Exercise of Critical Content

Circle the most correct answer.

1. Baby Sherman is being gavage fed. To check the placement of the tube, the nurse would:
   a. Measure the tube with the tube that was just removed.
   b. Insert only 6 inches of tube then pullback about 1/2 inch of tube.
   c. Aspirate gastric contents or listen to stomach with a stethoscope as 0.5 cc of air is insufflated.
   d. Loop the tube behind the infant's ear and measure to the umbilicus.

2. Joseph, a 35-week, 1580 gm male infant, was delivered to an 18-year-old primigravida. Joseph is demonstrating signs of respiratory distress. What is the first nursing action that should be taken?
   a. Notify the health care provider.
   b. Maintain a patent airway.
   c. If cyanosis occurs, provide oxygen.
   d. Apply monitoring electrodes.

3. Joesph's oxygen concentration is carefully regulated by watching his PO_2 levels because high blood levels of oxygen:
   a. Cause cardiac shunt closures, although the latter are not permanent.
   b. Cause peripheral circulatory collapse.
   c. May cause retinal spasms, leading to potential retrolental fibroplasia.
   d. May produce hyperbilirubinemia and severe jaundice.

4. Joseph does develop hyperbilirubinemia and is placed under phototherapy. The nurse will:
   a. Remove all of Joseph's clothing to expose all of his skin.
   b. Cover Joseph's eyes with patches to protect them from the light source.
   c. Observe Joseph for signs and symptoms of dehydration.
   d. All of the above are interventions the nurse must preform.

5. Infants of diabetic mothers are at risk for:
   a. Erythroblastosis fetalis.
   b. Hypercalcemia.
   c. Respiratory distress syndrome.
   d. Seizures.

6. Christopher is born with congenital syphilis. He most likely contracted it from his mother?
    a. At the time of birth.
    b. During the fifth month of pregnancy.
    c. During the second month of pregnancy.
    d. During the seventh month of pregnancy.

7. Sabrina was born with heroin addiction and is experiencing withdrawal symptoms. Nursing management for Sabrina include:
    a. Administration of methadone and frequent assessment of vital signs.
    b. Frequent assessment of vital signs and wrapping the infant snugly in a blanket.
    c. Meticulous skin and perineal care and frequent tactile stimulation.
    d. Minimal tactile stimulation and the provision of loose, nonrestrictive clothing.

8. Renold is a fetal alcohol syndrome infant. A symptom of this syndrome would be:
    a. Very poor feeder.
    b. Hypoactive nonnutritive suck reflex.
    c. Lethargy and long periods of sleep.
    d. Hypothermia because of lowered metabolic rate.

9. Describe a sign indicative of hypoglycemia in a newborn.
    a. Blotchy skin.
    b. Hypertonia.
    c. Jitteriness.
    d. Soft, weak cry.

10. The care of the high-risk infant by the parents should be initiated:
    a. Early and not just prior to the infant's discharge.
    b. At the time of the infant's discharge.
    c. When the nurse comes to visit the home after discharge.
    d. None of the above are correct.

Matching Exercise of Critical Content

Match the oxygen device or laboratory test with its purpose.

	Purpose	Oxygen device/Laboratory test
_____	1. Electrode attached to the infant's skin to measure the PaO$_2$ of blood flowing past the site.	A. Oxygen analyzer
_____	2. Device that measures the percentage of oxygen being delivered to the neonate.	B. Arterial blood gas analysis (ABG)
_____	3. Noninvasive method of measuring the oxygen saturation of arterial hemoglobin.	C. Transcutaneous oxygen monitoring (TC)
_____	4. 1 ml or less of blood is obtained directly from umbilical, temporal, brachial, or radial artery.	D. Pulse oximetry

True and False Exercise of Critical Content

The following statements require you to assess whether or not they are true or false. If the statement is false, rewrite it so that it is correct.

1. Potential complications for the high-risk newborn include oxygen toxicity, hyperbilirubinemia, and kernicterus. (True/False).

2. Nurses do not have to teach parents to perform therapies at home. (True/False).

3. Birth asphyxia is a high-risk condition characterized by hypoxemia, hypercarbia, and acidosis. (True/False).

4. With birth asphyxia, if immediate resuscitation is not begun, irreversible changes in brain and myocardial function will lead to permanent brain damage or death. (True/False).

5. The infant of a diabetic mother is often SGA. (True/False).

6. Universal body substance precautions are observed with every neonate to protect other newborns and staff members from transmission of the infection. (True/False).

7. One of the most serious complications for the neonate is intracranial hemorrhage. (True/False).

8. Rh incompatibility occurs when the mother is Rh positive and the fetus is Rh negative. (True/False).

Critical Thinking Exercise

1. Lynnette delivered a high-risk infant at 30 weeks gestation. The infant was transferred to a level III facility. Explain to Lynnette the functions of a Level III nursery. Compare the three levels of nurseries. Describe the education a nurse must obtain to work at each level.

2. Compare and contrast infants who are: LGA, AGA, SGA.

3. Generate a plan to prevent altered parenting for a neonate in the intensive care nursery.

CHAPTER 34

Congenital Anomalies in the Neonate

Overview

One of the most distressing situations health team members face is the birth of a neonate with a congenital anomaly. In most cases the anomaly was undiagnosed and unexpected. Defects may be missed even with ultrasonography. The birth attendant should inform the parents at once that there is a problem. This chapter discusses the most common abnormalities found and summarizes appropriate nursing care.

Learning Objectives

After studying the material in this chapter, the student will be able to:

- Discuss immediate care of the parents on the birth of a neonate with a congenital anomaly.
- Discuss legal and ethical dilemmas related to providing or withholding care to the newborn with a congenital defect.
- Identify the most common types of congenital anomalies detected in the neonatal period.
- Describe the physical characteristics of a neonate with Down syndrome.
- Explain the importance of screening for phenylketonuria.

Application of Key Terms

Match the definition in column two with the key terms in column one.

_____ 1. Anomaly   A. Present at birth.
_____ 2. Atresia   B. Genetically transmitted from parent to offspring.
_____ 3. Cogenital   C. Marked deviation from the norm.
_____ 4. Hereditary   D. Congenital absence or closure of a normal body opening.

CONGENITAL ANOMALIES IN THE NEONATE

Short Answer Exercise of Critical Content

1. Write the appropriate terminology for the following acronyms:

   a. ASD:

   b. VSD:

   c. PDA:

   d. PKU:

   e. MSUD:

2. Baby Emily is screened for PKU at 10 days of age. Results are elevated and further testing confirms classic phenylketonuria. The mother is notified by the health care provider and a referral is made to the local genetic center for follow-up dietary management. Provide answers to the following questions the mother asks.

   a. "Would my diet have affected the results since I am breastfeeding?"

   b. "Will my baby be retarded?"

   c. "Does this mean my baby is allergic to milk?"

3. Provide the rationale for positioning a newborn with myelomeningocele on his/her side.

4. List the rationale for aspiration of gastric contents from the child with diaphragmatic hernia.

5. Indicate the rationale for frequent turning and positioning of an infant with pulmonary agenesis.

UNIT V: ADAPTATION IN THE POSTPARTUM PERIOD

6. Provide the rationale for giving the parents of a child with a major congenital anomaly a picture of the infant prior to transporting him/her to a Level III center.

7. Indicate the rationale for serial measurements of the abdomen of an infant with bilious vomiting.

Multiple Choice Exercise of Critical Content

Circle the most correct answer.

1. An outpouching of the meninges and cerebrospinal fluid through a defect in the vertebral column is know as:
    a. Spina bifida occult.
    b. Hydrocephalus.
    c. Anencephaly.
    d. Meningocele.

2. Lisa was born at 36 weeks gestation. She has a scaphoid-shape abdomen and bowel sounds can be heard over the chest wall. Prior to emergency surgery, she must be watched closely for:
    a. Motor and sensory function.
    b. Bulging, tense fontanelles.
    c. Asphyxia and respiratory distress.
    d. Cyanosis with feedings.

3. Infants with congenital heart disease may be gavage fed to:
    a. Make the feeding easier for the nursing staff.
    b. Decrease energy requirements and prevent infant fatigue.
    c. Make sure the infant gets a specified amount of feeding.
    d. Keep the infant on a rigid feeding schedule.

4. Sandra planned to breastfeed but baby Heather was born with a cleft lip. Sandra should be encouraged to:
    a. Pump her breast because surgical repair can be done soon after birth and breastfeeding initiated.
    b. Give up the idea of breastfeeding and switch to exclusively feeding by bottle.
    c. Learn to gavage feed Heather because she will have to be fed this way the rest of her life.
    d. Learn how to use a Brecht feeder because Heather cannot swallow breastmilk.

CONGENITAL ANOMALIES IN THE NEONATE

5. Joey was born with his abdominal contents protruding through a defect in the ventral abdominal wall. This is know as:

   a. Pyloric stenosis.

   b. Exstrophy of the bladder.

   c. Omphalocele.

   d. Hydrocephalus.

6. Gerri just delivered a baby that has been diagnosed with Down syndrome. A major nursing intervention at this time is:

   a. To prevent Gerri from bonding with the baby.

   b. Demonstrate foot exercises Gerri should perform three times a day on the baby.

   c. Support Gerri and help her work through the grieving process.

   d. Teach Gerri all she will need to know to care for the infant so that a referral will not be necessary.

Matching Exercise of Critical Content

Match the following cardiac anomalies with the appropriate category, **A**; cyanotic heart disease or **B**; acyonotic heart disease.

_____ 1. Atrial septal defect.

_____ 2. Tetralogy of Fallot.

_____ 3. Coarctation of the aorta.

_____ 4. Transposition of the great vessels.

_____ 5. Patent ductus arteriosus.

_____ 6. Ventricular septal defect.

_____ 7. Pulmonary stenosis.

True and False Exercise of Critical Content

The following statements require you to assess whether or not they are true or false. If the statement is false, rewrite it so that it is correct.

1. When an infant has anomalous venous return, one or more pulmonary veins empty into the right atrium. (True/False).

2. Most infants with pyloric stenosis begin to vomit immediately after birth. (True/False).

3. In gastroschisis, the defect is most commonly located to the left of the umbilical cord. (True/False).

4. Patent urachus is the persistence of a normal fetal anatomical structure. (True/False).

5. Following the birth of an infant with a congenital anomaly, it is normal for parents to experience reactions similar to the grieving process. (True/False).

6. Hydrocephalus is rarely associated with myelomeningocele. (True/False).

7. The neonate is an obligate nose breather. (True/False).

8. A right-to-left shunting of blood occurs in the presence of patent ductus arteriosus. (True/False).

9. Humans are born with 48 chromosomes. (True/False).

10. Neonatal screening tests can detect congenital hypothyroidism. (True/False).

Critical Thinking Exercise

1. Analyze different factors which may influence the impact that the birth of a child with a major birth defect has on a family. Critique how these factors may affect family dynamics.

2. Produce a list of support groups in your area for parents experiencing the birth of a child with major birth defect. Recommend national organizations that lend support and/or information to these families.

3. Many legal and ethical issues are involved when a newborn has a congenital defect. Specify strategies that the neonatal nurse can use to deal effectively with legal and ethical dilemmas.

CHAPTER 35

Maternal and Infant Nutrition

Overview

New mothers often are motivated to return to their nonpregnant physical state as guickly as possible and are open to suggestions about nutrition and exercise to expedite the process. Mothers who choose to breastfeed require special support and teaching as they learn the necessary skills. The postpartum nurse is able to assess the concerns, eating habits, and activities of new mothers. This chapter provides the information necessary to assess and plan appropriate nursing actions to meet the nutritional needs of women and their neonates.

Learning Objectives

After studying the material in this chapter, the student will be able to:

- Explain the nutritional requirements of the lactating and nonlactating mother during the fourth trimester.
- Discuss the effects of nutrition on the quality and quantity of breast milk produced.
- Explain the nutritional requirements of the infant from birth to 6 months of age.
- Identify factors that affect maternal weight loss after childbirth.
- Advise mothers about dietary recommendations for themselves and their infants during the fourth trimester.

Application of Key Terms

Match the definitions in column two with the key terms in column one.

_____ 1. Casein

_____ 2. Colostrum

_____ 3. Epidermal growth factor

_____ 4. Fluoride

_____ 5. Lactalbumin

_____ 6. Lactation

_____ 7. Renal solute load

_____ 8. Whey

A. Liquid that remains after the cream and curd are separated from the milk.

B. Postpartum production of milk.

C. Important constituent of whey.

D. Breast fluid secreted 2 or 3 days after childbirth and before the onset of true lactation.

E. Metabolic end products, especially nitrogenous compounds and electrolytes, that must be excreted by the kidneys.

F. The principal protein present in milk curds.

G. A dietary mineral necessary for the development of dental enamel.

H. A polypeptide found in breast milk with growth-promoting activity.

MATERNAL AND INFANT NUTRITION

Short Answer Exercise of Critical Content

1. Allyson, a new mother, states she wishes to breastfeed her infant and asks you why breast-feeding might be better than formula feeding. Explain the benefits of breastfeeding.

2. Angela is very concerned about her baby's formula needs during the first year of life. Explain to her how and when formula needs increase.

3. Determine what should be included in the diet of a lactating mother.

4. List four criteria that would be appropriate to use in evaluating whether or not an infant has been well-nourished.

    a.

    b.

    c.

    d.

Multiple Choice Exercise of Critical Content

Circle the most correct answer.

1. Nadine is breastfeeding and asks you how she can tell if the baby is getting enough. Your best reply would be:
    a. There is no way to tell. You just need to keep feeding him.
    b. If the baby sleeps 3-4 hours between each feeding and is wetting at least six diapers a day he's getting enough.
    c. You must keep giving 2-3 ounces of water after every breast feeding to make sure he gets enough.
    d. You need to express your milk and measure it so you will know the exact amount.

2. Nadine asks when she should begin feeding her baby solid foods. You inform her that breast milk is sufficient to meet most of the nutritional needs for:

   a. The first month of life.//
   b. The first 2 to 3 months.//
   c. The first 4 to 6 months.//
   d. The first year of life.

3. Nadine is concerned about the weight she has gained during pregnancy and wants to go on a diet. You would advise her to:

   a. Begin a strict diet and exercise program immediately.//
   b. Limit her fluid intake to reduce the possibility for retention.//
   c. Eliminate all carbohydrates from her diet to help her lose weight.//
   d. Avoid trying to lose weight until she weans her infant from the breast.

Matching Exercise of Critical Content

Match the following comments with the category of A: Breastfeeding or B: Cow's milk.

_____ 1. Protein more easily digested.

_____ 2. 80% of protein in form of casein.

_____ 3. Whey constitutes 60% of protein.

_____ 4. Higher in calcium.

_____ 5. Carbohydrate content is 4.8%.

_____ 6. Rich source of cholesterol.

True and False Exercise of Critical Content

The following statements require you to assess whether or not they are true or false. If the statement is false, rewrite it so that it is correct.

1. Breastfeeding increased significantly during the 1970s, peaked in the early 1980s and has remained the same. (True/False).

2. Infant suckling stimulates the productions of oxytocin, which causes the uterus to contract, thereby promoting good uterine tone. (True/False).

MATERNAL AND INFANT NUTRITION

3. The lactating woman needs extra fluid and should drink a minimum of 2 liters of fluid per day. (True/False).

4. The formula-feeding mother does not have special dietary needs. (True/False).

Critical Thinking Exercise

1. Detect how breast milk of poorly nourished populations differ from that of well-nourished groups. Propose what implications this has for infant growth.

2. Generate a list of the ethnic and cultural groups in your area. Working with a group of fellow students, develop teaching materials appropriate to each group. Produce adequate information on the following topics: lactation diet, non-lactating postpartal diet, breastfeeding information, formula preparation and feeding, adding solid food to infant s diet, and weaning.

CHAPTER 36

Individual and Family Adaptation in the Year After Childbirth

Overview

Ongoing adaptations are required of families during the first year of life with an infant. Changes occur in roles, communication among family members, family health practices, and family-community interactions. The primary goal of nursing care of new families is to facilitate achievement of developmental tasks and support the complex adjustments required. This chapter discusses family adaptations during the first year of an infant's life and describes effective nursing care to promote a positive and healthy transition.

Learning Objectives

After studying the material in this chapter, the student will be able to:

- Describe changing roles in families during the year after childbirth.
- Describe unanticipated stressors encountered by families during the year after childbirth.
- Discuss myths about parenthood.
- Relate family characteristics to ease transition to the parental role.
- Assess family adaptation.
- Identify nursing objectives for families during the year after childbirth.
- Identify families at risk for difficulties in adaptation.
- Describe nursing actions that facilitate healthy family adaptation.
- Develop teaching care plans that foster self-care in the family during the year after childbearing.

UNIT V: ADAPTATION IN THE POSTPARTUM PERIOD 225

Application of Key Terms

Match the definitions in column two with the key terms in column one.

_____ 1. Blended family
_____ 2. Behavioral cues
_____ 3. Colic
_____ 4. Failure to thrive (nonorganic)
_____ 5. Family development
_____ 6. Irritable infant syndrome
_____ 7. Role taking

A. Assuming a pattern of behavior that is socially assigned or adopted.
B. Abdominal pain that occurs in infants, principally during the first few months.
C. Infants who not only fail to gain weight but also may lose it.
D. Also known as colic.
E. The developmental task of incorporating the new family member into the preexisting family unit.
F. Signs that indicate the parents are attaching with the infant.
G. When parents remarry and then have a child.

Short Answers Exercise of Critical Content

1. _____ is the natural beginning of all human relationships and the first stage of the attachment process.

2. The neonate has a unique personality or _____.

3. Colic may disrupt family functioning. Characteristics of colic include:

   a.

   b.

   c.

   d.

   e.

   f.

4. Identify five behavioral characteristics in a newborn that could negatively affect parental-infant interaction.

   a.

   b.

   c.

   d.

   e.

5. Child abuse is universal and crosses all cultural and socioeconomic barriers. List and briefly define four types of abuse.

   a.

   b.

   c.

   d.

Multiple Choice Exercise of Critical Content

Circle the most correct answer.

1. After delivery you observe the new father intently staring at his newborn while he is holding him. The father is lightly running his finger tips over the baby's face. The father is beginning:

   a. Parenting.
   b. Discipline.
   c. Acquaintance.
   d. Development.

UNIT V: ADAPTATION IN THE POSTPARTUM PERIOD 227

2. Every time you go into Leslie s postpartum room she asks the same questions about baby care. Leslie is:

   a. Seeking validation.

   b. A very poor mother.

   c. Demonstrating failure to thrive.

   d. Testing the nursing staff.

3. Dawn has a two-year-old daughter at home and has just delivered a son. She asks what she can do to prevent sibling rivalry. Your best answer might be:

   a. Leave them alone together in a room so they can get used to each other.

   b. Punish your daughter for any signs of regression and not being a good big sister .

   c. Arrange time for the daughter and you alone and include her in as much care for the infant you can.

   d. Send the daughter to live with her grandparents for at least the first week.

4. Hurang is from China and rejects the nurses plans to bring the newborn to the health care provider before its seventh day of life to repeat the PKU. Hurang s reasons are based on:

   a. She is a neglectful mother and will not seek health care for the infant.

   b. The first month after birth is time for confinement and rest.

   c. She will be back at work and will be unable to arrange time off.

   d. The baby will not be available because it will be sent to live with it grandparents.

Matching Exercise of Critical Content

Match the following terms relating to parental role taking with their correct definition. Some terms may be used more than once.

Definitions:	Parental role taking terms:
____ 1. Awareness of the unique characteristics of their infant.	A. Emotional involvement
____ 2. Differentiation of infant as separate person from mother.	B. Acquaintance
	C. Individualization
____ 3. Rapid precess occurring immediately after birth reflecting parent to infant attachment.	D. Bonding
____ 4. Feeling of significance of infant in parents lives.	E. Attachment
	F. Acceptance
____ 5. Gathering information about actual infant and comparing to expected newborn.	
____ 6. Integration of emotional involvement and individualization accepted without reservation.	
____ 7. Reciprocal relationship between the parent and infant that grows during first year.	
____ 8. Basis for attachment; reinforces expectations or changes from expectations.	

True and False Exercise of Critical Content

The following statements require you to assess whether or not they are true or false. If the statement is false, rewrite it so that it is correct.

1. The physical and emotional survival of the infant depends on accomplishment of the parent-infant attachment process, which is a major developmental task to be accomplished in the first year. (True/False).

2. Women attain the maternal role by gaining competence as a caregiver and nurturing parent. (True/False).

3. All families function the same and should be treated the same. (True/False).

4. Two factor that can profoundly affect the health and well-being of childbearing families are postpartum depression and child abuse. (True/False).

Critical Thinking Exercise

1. You have been asked to teach a prenatal class about sibling rivalry. Formulate ideas to present that will assist with integrating the new baby into the family.

2. Allyson comes to the health care provider with sleep deprivation. Through questioning you learn that the baby is suffering from colic. Propose interventions to Allyson to assist with this troublesome time.

Answer Key

ANSWERS TO CHAPTER 1

Key terms

1. D; 2. E; 3. B; 4. A; 5. C; 6. F

Short answers

1. Possible answers include:

    Obstetric forceps by Peter Chamberlen (1560-1631)

    Modified by William Smellie (1697-1763)

    "Childbed" fever described as an epidemic by Francois Mauriceau (1637-1709).

    Spread of "childbed" fever by physicians hands discovered by Semmelweis

    Hegar's sign (softening of the lower segment of the uterus during pregnancy)

    Nagel's rule (a method for calculating estimated dates of birth).

2. Possible answers include:

    a. Federal funding for hospital construction - provided a centralized setting for physicians to practice.

    b. The increasing organization of medicine - the approach to childbirth became more technological.

    c. The popularity of analgesia for childbirth - contributed to physician control over maternity care.

    d. Advances in analgesia, anesthesia, operative and life-support techniques - these had to be done in the hospital, and by physicians.

    e. Legislation passed in many states outlawing midwifery - supported the belief that hospital-based care was superior.

    f. Economic pressures of the Great Depression of the 1930s - resulted in a sharp decline in the birth rate.

3. Social and economic factors

    Cost containment

    Cost of high technology

    Costs and appropriate use of intensive care

    Prospective payment.

Multiple-choice

1. c;   2. b;   3. c

Matching

1. C;   2. A;   3. E;   4. B, F;   5. D, F

True and False

1. True.

2. False.

    While some proponents of sibling participation feel that family bonding is increased and sibling rivalry may be lessened when the older child is present at the birth, studies have not conclusively proved this.

3. False.

    No studies have documented harmful effects of sibling participation in the birth experience.

4. True.

ANSWERS TO CHAPTER 2

Application of key terms

1. E;   2. C;   3. D;   4. H;   5. B;   6. A;   7. G;
8. F

Short answer

1. The nursing process provides a systematic approach to perinatal nursing care. The process focuses the nurse's attention on a logical progression of decisions and actions aimed at resolving specific health problems.

2. Possible Nursing Diagnoses .

    a. Constipation related to physiologic changes of pregnancy and iron supplementation.

    b. Knowledge deficit related to lack of experience in caring for a newborn.

    c. Altered nutrition (Less than body requirements) related to nausea and vomiting in pregnancy.

    d. Ineffective family coping related to parental role overload in caring for triplets.

3. The nurse plans and implements teaching based on the following considerations:

   Learning needs of the woman and her family members.

   Principles of teaching and learning.

   Physiologic and psychological condition of the woman, her neonate, and the family.

   Sociocultural factors.

Multiple choice

1. d;   2. c;   3. d

ANSWERS TO CHAPTER 3

Application of key terms

1. C;   2. E;   3. H;   4. G;   5. B;   6. F;   7. D;'
8. A

Short answers

1. There is concern about rising rates of low and very low birth weight infants among African Americans and other minorities in the United States. Adolescent pregnancies are increasing more rapidly among African Americans and are at more risk for low birth weight. Maternal well-being is also poorer among African American women. Hispanic American women tend to receive less prenatal care than the total population. Maternal and infant health indicators vary largely by socioeconomic status and acculturation. Diabetes, obesity and infectious diseases tend to be more prevalent in minority groups. Statistics on maternal and infant mortality indicate that individuals least able to afford private care have the worst obstetric and neonatal outcomes.

2. Barriers to optimal maternity care include:

   a. poverty

   b. discrimination

   c. impaired access to care

3. Association of Women's Health, Obstetric, and Neonatal Nurses (AWHONN)

4.
- a. The Certified Nurse Midwife.

    A registered nurse who has completed a certificate program or master's degree level educational program recognized by the American College of Nurse Midwifery. CNMs are prepared to deliver normal gynecologic care and primary care to women during pregnancy and childbirth. They can assume care of women and their newborns during the postbirth period. They manage labor and birth, prescribe, and perform certain medical and surgical procedures. They collaborate with physicians in the care of women with complex health problems.

- b. The Clinical Nurse Specialist

    A registered nurse who has completed a master's degree program in nursing. Specialized education includes reproductive health and expertise in planning supervision, and delivery of nursing care to families during the childbearing period. Major responsibilities are consultation, family and staff education, and coordination and delivery of nursing care to families requiring intensive nursing support.

- c. The Nurse Practitioner in Women's Health

    A registered nurse with advanced clinical preparation in the provision of primary care to women. This clinical preparation may be obtained in a certificate program or as part of a master's degree in nursing. States often require completion of a certification examination. NPs conduct comprehensive health assessments and manage normal prenatal, postbirth, and gynecologic care in collaboration with physicians and nurse midwives. They diagnose and treat common problems and refer women to physicians according to established protocols.

- d. Nurse Consultants

    Nurse consultants are experts in a particular area of practice who establish a private practice to provide consultation to agencies on a fee-for-service basis. They provide expert review of materials and act as expert witnesses in regard to potential professional liability issues. They also help develop equipment or products to be used in patient care. These roles require considerable clinical expertise as well as specialized skills and experience.

- e. The Nurse Scientist in Perinatal Nursing

    Nurse scientists are employed by schools of nursing, health care agencies, and government. They usually function in teaching, administration, and or research activities. The desired educational preparation is the doctoral degree. Nurse scientists in perinatal nursing are engaged in the study of health problems facing women and their families.

Multiple Choice

1. b;   2. c;   3. d

True and False

1. False.

    A court-ordered cesarean delivery can be obtained to protect the fetus.

2. True

3. False.

Both risks and benefits to the fetus and woman must be taken into consideration.

ANSWERS TO CHAPTER 4

Key terms

1. D; 2. I; 3. L; 4. F; 5. C; 6. B; 7. H;
8. M; 9. K; 10. G; 11. O; 12. J; 13. N; 14. A;
15. E

Short answers

1. Seventh and 14th week of development

    12 weeks

    Testosterone

2. The chief functions of the testes are to produce viable sperm and the male hormone testosterone.

3. The penis.

4. Corpora cavernosa

    tunica albuginea

    corpus spongiosum

5. Glans penis

6. The epididymis is the beginning part of the excretory duct of each testis and stores sperm.

7. Prostate—Surrounds the neck of the bladder and secretes a thin, opalescent fluid into the urethra.

    Bulbourethral (Cowper's) Glands—Located in the urogenital diaphragm and secrete a clear, viscous, and alkaline fluid to help neutralize the acidic female vaginal secretions.

8. Vaginal orifice and clitoris.

9. 4 cm.; paraurethral

10. Perineum

11.
   a. excretory duct of the uterus
   b. female organ of copulation
   c. canal for the vaginal birth of a baby

12. 4.0 to 5.0

13.

Ligament	Location	Function
Broad Ligament	Wing like transverse fold of peritoneum that arises from the floor of the pelvic cavity between the bladder and the rectum.	Divides the pelvic cavity into anterior and posterior sections providing support to the uterus, ovaries and tubes.
Round Ligament	Arises below and anteriorly to the oviducts. Extends from the broad ligament throught the inguinal canal and terminates within the upper portion of the labia majora.	Extends from either side of the lateral portions of the uterus to support the uterus.
Uterosacral Ligament	Attaches to the cervix and encircles the rectum.	Forms the lateral boundries of the rectouterine cul-de-sac and supports the uterus.

14.
   a. secretes the female hormone estrogen
   b. produces the midcycle spurt of estrogen necessary for ovulation
   c. becomes the corpus luteum if pregnancy occurs
   d. corpus luteum produces estrogen and progesterone

15. Estrogen; progesterone; FSH; LH.

   a. Satisfaction of sexual desires
   b. Maturation of the reproductive organs
   c. Preparation of the reproductive organs for conception, gestation, and childbirth

Multiple Choice

1. b;   2. c;   3. d;   4. c;   5. c;   6. b;   7. c;
8. c

ANSWERS TO CHAPTER 5

Matching

1. C, F;   2. A, H;   3. D, I;   4. B, J, L;   5. E, G, K

True/False

1. True
2. False.

   Sexual sensations pass through the pudendal nerve, the sacral plexus, the sacral portion of the spinal cord, and up the spinal cord to areas of the cerebrum.

3. False.

   The fibers are called tunica dartos.

4. False.

   The prostate gland secretes an alkaline opalescent fluid and does not store sperm.

5. True

ANSWERS TO CHAPTER 5

Key Terms

1. D;   2. B;   3. H;   4. G;   5. E;   6. A;   7. C;
8. I;   9. F.

Short Answers

1.
   a. Excitement phase. The primary reaction to sexual stimuli is vasocongestion. This may be triggered by direct physical stimulation, sight, or erotic train of thought. The second reaction is myotonia, spasms in the hands and feet, facial grimaces, and tensing of extremities or other parts of the body.
   b. Plateau phase. Characterized by a degree of sexual arousal that is much higher than the excitement phase and is lower than the threshold level required to trigger orgasm.
   c. Orgasm phase. A reflex response to a stimulus that is sufficiently effective to reach the threshold level of arousal. Muscles contract and ejaculation occurs in this phase.
   d. Resolution phase. The return of the genital organs and body to the unaroused state.

2. Labia majora: Flatten and separate away from vaginal opening.

   Labia minora: Increase 2 to 3 times in size and deepen in color.

   Clitoris: becomes engorged. Shortens and withdraws under labial or clitoral hood near end of plateau; may be very sensitive.

   Pelvic muscles: Various muscle fibers, muscles, and groups of muscles contract in a spasm.

   Vagina: Lubrication is due to vasocongestion and occurs within 10-30 sec. of the onset of stimulation. The diameter of the vaginal opening is reduced with engorgement at the Plateau phase. Inner two-thirds of vagina lengthens and distends during orgasm.

   Cervix and uterus: The uterus and cervix elevate and pull the cervix out of the way.

   Breast: Erection of nipples due to contraction of muscle fibers. Areola may become engorged. Breast may become engorged. Breast may increase in size.

3. Penis: Vasocongestion in the penis causes erection and lengthening.

   Scrotum and testes: Scrotum thickens, flattens, and elevates. Testes enlarge and elevate.

   Prostate: Seminal fluid collects in prostatic urethra.

   Seminal vesicles: Contract to release fluid and sperm.

   Cowper's glands: Secrets small amount of clear fluid called preejaculatory fluid. May contain live spermatozoa.

   Pelvic muscles: Muscle tension in both involuntary and voluntary muscles occur.

Multiple Choice

1. d; 2. a; 3. d; 4. c; 5. b; 6. b.

True and False

1. False.

   Correct anatomical names should be used.

2. False.

   Children learn about their sexuality in infancy

3. True.
4. False.

   By age nine to twelve, children should know what body changes to expect at puberty.

5. True.

ANSWERS TO CHAPTER 6 237

6. True.
7. True.
8. True.
9. True.
10. False.

Breastfeeding is **NOT** considered effective because the pattern of hormonal changes is unpredictable.

ANSWERS TO CHAPTER 6

Key terms

1. B;   2. F;   3. E;   4. G;   5. J;   6. A;   7. C;
8. D;   9. H;   10. I

Short answers

1.
   a. Coronary heart disease
   b. Cancer of the lung and reproductive organs
   c. Accidental injury
   d. Eating disorders
   e. STDs especially AIDS

2. Screening for breast cancer includes breast self-examination (BSE) and periodic screening with mammography and clinical breast examination by a health professional. Guidelines for breast cancer screening are:

   - BSE monthly
   - Annual breast examination by a health care professional
   - Baseline mammogram between ages 35 and 40
   - Mammogram every 1-2 years for women between the ages of 40 and 50, every year thereafter.

3. The major tool in the early diagnosis of cervical cancer is the Papanicolaou (Pap) smear. The Pap smear is a screening test that identifies precancerous or cancerous changes in cervical cells.

   The American Cancer Society advises that all sexually active women receive a Pap smear annually. After having a normal Pap smear for 2 consecutive years, a woman should have a Pap smear every 3 years until age 65.

4. Anorexia is a condition of extreme weight loss because of inadequate food intake, and is defined as weight loss to a level of 15% or more below expected weight for height and age.

   Bulimia is characterized by episodes of binge eating (eating of extraordinarily large amounts of food) and the subsequent use of self-induced vomiting, cathartics, laxatives, diuretics, and over-exercise to control body weight.

   Anorexia - middle class, European Americans; preadolescents

   Bulimia - Adolescents

5. Progestin, endometrial hyperplasia and endometrial carcinoma.

6. Possible answers include

   Keep genital area dry by wearing 100% cotton underwear

   Avoid clothing that is tight in the crotch

   Sleep without underwear

   Always wipe from front to back

   Change sanitary napkins and tampons frequently

   Practice safe sex through abstinence or use of condoms

   Report any suspicious discharge, pain, or irritation to the physician immediately

7.

Disease	Treatment	Diagnosis
Chlamydia	Cervical culture	Tetracycline or doxycycline
Herpes	Clinical symptoms Pap smear ELISA	No cure Oral acyclovir or topical ointment
Trichomoniasis	Wet mount Pap smear	Metronidazole vinegar douches
Condyloma	Clinical appearance	Laser therapy, topical podophyllin
Gonorrhea	Cultures from urethra, cervix, or rectum	Ceftriaxone Penicillin Amoxicillin Ampicillin
Syphilis	Blood tests, VDRL, RPR, FTA-ABS	Penicillin
HIV/AIDS	ELISA	None or AZT

ANSWERS TO CHAPTER 7

Multiple choice

1. b; 2. c; 3. d; 4. d; 5. b; 6. a

Matching

1. F; 2. D; 3. E; 4. G; 5. A; 6. C;
7. B; 8. I; 9. J; 10. K; 11. H

ANSWERS TO CHAPTER 7

Key terms

1. D; 2. J; 3. O; 4. Q; 5. N; 6. R; 7. E;
8. H; 9. R; 10. S; 11. G; 12. K; 13. A; 14. U;
15. C; 16. B; 17. T; 18. I; 19. L; 20. M; 21. F.

Short answers

1. Possible answers include:

    easy to use

    noninterruptive

    total safety

    total effectiveness

    low expense

    no side effects

    availability with minimum health care provider contact

    instant reversibility

2.
    A. severe abdominal pain

    C. Chest pain or shortness of breath

    H. severe headache

    E. eye problems

    S. severe leg pain

3.
- P. pain-abdominal, pelvic, with intercourse
- A. abnormal bleeding
- I. infection (vaginal discharge, fever, chills)
- N. no period
- S. strings absent

ANSWERS TO CHAPTER 7

4.

	Advantages	**Disadvantages**
Diaphragm	a. nonhormonal, very safe, may offer protection against STDS.	b. Interruptive, messy, much motivation required, some increase in bladder infection, requires medical contact.
Cervical Cap	c. Same as diaphragm. Can remain in place 48 hours.	d. Same as diaphragm, however may not be as messy. May be difficult to remove.
Sponges	e. Same as diaphragm. Works up to 24 hours.	f. Same as diaphragm. May increase risk of T.S.S. May tear requiring pelvic exam for removal. May cause allergic reaction.
Vaginal Pouch	g. Additional female-controlled contraceptive choice. Protection against bacterial and viral STDs.	h. Allergy to the material or discomfort from the rings might occur.
Condoms	i. No prescription needed, safe, STD protection, man's responsibility.	j. Interruptive, may be irritating.
Foams, Jellies	k. No prescription needed, safe, protects from STDs.	l. Interruptive, messy, requires motivation, may be irritating.
Oral Contraceptives	m. Noninterruptive, highly effective, may have lighter menses with fewer cramps, less PID, less anemia.	n. Expensive, requires prescription and medical contact, irregular menses, cardiovascular complications.
Norplant	o. Noninterruptive, effective up to 5 years, no risk to fetus, highly effective, new.	p. No protection against STDs, surgical complications infections at insertion sites, removal may become difficult.
IUD	q. Noninterruptive, highly effective, user doesn't need to remember to do something, not a drug.	r. Increased risk of PID, ectopic pregnancy, increased menstrual bleeding and cramping, requires medical contact.
Sterilization	s. Highly effective, no side effects, considered permanent.	t. Frequently an irreversible surgical procedure, vasectomy does not provide instant sterility.

5.
   a. Calendar method - fertile period is calculated on the basis of the longest and shortest of the 8 most recent menstrual cycles.
   b. BBT method - fertile period (ovulation) is designated in retrospect by the occurrence of a biphasic temperature pattern.
   c. Cervical Mucus method - fertility is determined on basis of cyclical changes in the characteristics of the cervical mucus.
   d. Symptothermal method - fertility is determined by using all of the preceding methods.

6.
   a. Primary infertility
   b. Secondary infertility
   c. Situational infertility

7.
   a. Ovarian Factors - - 15%
   b. Tubal Factors - - 25-50% from Chlamydra

   PID 10-20%; with three episodes of infection, 55-75%
   c. Cervical Factors - - 5-10%

8.
   a. Sperm Abnormalities - - unknown %

   Varicocele - - 20-40%

9.
   a. Semen analysis to determine involvement of a male factor; hysterosalpingogram to determined tubal patency in view of previous history; BBT or endometrial biopsy to determine adequacy of luteal phase.
   b. Possible treatment options: (1) If a male factor is found it will need to be investigated by urologist; possible treatments would be surgical correction of underlying cause or artificial insemination with donor sperm; (2) If a tubal factor is found surgical correction might be an option or form of invitro fertilization; (3) If an inadequate luteal phase is found (or other ovulatory problems) pharmacological therapy would be considered.

ANSWERS TO CHAPTER 7

10.

Procedure	Parameter(s) Assessed	Description
Semen analysis	a. Assesses sperm count, motility, morphology.	b. Man produces a masturbated specimen after 48-72 hours of abstinence.
Sims-Huhner Test	c. Assesses cervical mucus characteristics at ovulation and receptivity to sperm, and sperm-mucus interaction.	d. Woman is examined within 8 hours of having intercourse on the day of anticipated ovulation.
BBT Chart	e. Assesses occurrence of ovulation and adequacy of luteal phase.	f. Temperature is taken before arising each morning looking for a biphasic pattern.
Hysterosalpingogram	g. Assess tubal and uterine structure and patency.	h. Radiopaque dye is injected through the cervix, its flow through the uterus and tubes is radiologically observed.
Endometrial Biopsy	i. Assesses occurrence of ovulation and adequacy of secretory tissue for implantation to occur.	j. Endometrial tissue is obtained on day 21 of the menstrual cycle and microscopically examined for progesterone effect.

Multiple Choice

1. b;   2. a;   3. c;   4. c;   5. d;   6. b;   7. b;
8. c;   9. a;   10. c;   11. c;   12. b

Matching

1. B, D, E, F, H;   2. A, B, D, E, G, H;   3. C, D, E, F, H.

True or False

1. False.

   The legal system is rather undecided and at this time, the gestational mother's rights are subordinate to the genetic mother.

2. True

3. False.

The procedures are very complex and may induce stress, fatigue, or a sense of isolation.

4. False.

A study reported a decrease in mastery over life, self-esteem, and support.

5. True.
6. True.

ANSWERS TO CHAPTER 8

Key terms

1. E;   2. C;   3. H;   4. F;   5. A;   6. D;   7. B;
8. I;   9. G

Short answers

1. Preparing to provide for the physical care of the expected baby.

    Adapting financial patterns to meet increasing needs.

    Defining evolving role patterns.

    Expanding communication to meet present and future emotional needs.

    Reorienting relationships with relatives.

2. Maternal developmental tasks might include:

    a. the pregnancy.
    b. Establishing a relationship with the unborn child.
    c. Adjusting to changes in self.
    d. Adjusting to changes in the couple relationship.
    e. Preparing for birth and early parenthood.

3. Paternal tasks of pregnancy might include:

    The paternal tasks of pregnancy are similar psychological since he does not experience the biologically inducted changes the woman does.

ANSWERS TO CHAPTER 8

4. Psychosocial/cultural factors that might be included are:

    a. A value of children.
    b. Number of children desired.
    c. Correct age for childbearing.
    d. Acceptability of extramarital sexual activity.
    e. Acceptability of pregnancy outside of marriage.
    f. Appropriate male and female behavior.
    g. Availability and acceptability of contraception.
    h. Peer and family pressures toward or away from parenthood.

5. Psychosocial/cultural assessments that might be included are:

    a. Woman's age and level of development.
    b. Socioeconomic status.
    c. Financial support for this pregnancy and other health care needs.
    d. Is this pregnancy desired?
    e. Is pregnancy viewed as a health or illness state?
    f. Type of family support for the pregnancy.
    g. Who makes decisions about pregnancy and health care?
    h. Is pregnancy supported by peer group?
    i. What special diet is needed by pregnancy? Are there foods to be avoided?
    j. Are there special activities that need to be done during pregnancy? Are there activities that need to be avoided?

6. After determining that the woman is not in active labor, get an interpreter to talk with her and, get informed consent for this induction procedure. Find out who the child is and if there is someone else available to care for the child.

7. Assess what language she speaks best. Determine her ability to read, write, and speak English. Face her, speak slowly in a normal tone of voice. If talking does not work, show her equipment, show procedure on self or another, use gestures/actions to explain. Try printing what is wanted. Draw or point to pictures. Make flash cards illustrating words or phrases from a dictionary. Point to words in a dual language dictionary. Get an interpreter.

Multiple-choice

1. d;   2. d;   3. c;   4. c;   5. b;   6. a

Matching

1. E;   2. C;   3. D;   4. A;   5. B

1. G;   2. A;   3. C;   4. B;   5. F;   6. E;   7. D;
8. H

True and False

1. True
2. False.
   The study identified four different levels of awareness.
3. False.
   They are in a large part products of society, socioeconomic class, and culture.
4. True.
5. False.
   Pregnancy is a time of increased vulnerability to crisis.

ANSWERS TO CHAPTER 9

Keys terms

1. C;   2. E;   3. A;   4. D;   5. B;   6. F

ANSWERS TO CHAPTER 9

Short answers

1. Early Adolescence: (a) Rapid, peak height attained, (b) Preoccupation with physical changes; requires frequent reworking of image; preoccupation with appearance, (c) Peers, (d) Concrete operations; here and now orientation; egocentric, (e) Strained by early striving for independence, (f) Some sex orientation; crushes on adult role models; telephonitis.

    Middle Adolescence: (g) Adult height and body proportions usually completed at this time. (h) Stabilizing with achievement of adult physical stature, (i) Peer group importance recedes; relationships with fewer, close individuals, (j) Formal operations; generation of options to solve problems; regression to egocentric here and now methods when under stress, (k) Struggles over emancipation continue, (l) Begins heterosexual activity; sexual experimentation ranging from kissing to petting and intercourse; absence of true psychological intimacy.

    Late Adolescence: (m) Physical growth complete, (n) Stable, (o) Peer group importance recedes; relationships with fewer, close individuals, (p) Abstract, with future orientation, (q) Assumed adult to adult quality; fewer issues over independence, (r) Characterized by mutuality and reciprocity, caring for another; loss of narcissistic orientation.

2. Answers might include:

    a. Socioeconomic status.
    b. Early sexual activity.
    c. Perceived limited life opportunities.
    d. Family characteristics.
    e. Developmental status.
    f. Substance use and abuse.

3.
    a. Many adolescents deny, ignore, or incorrectly interpret the signs of pregnancy.
    b. Inadequate prenatal care.

4. Answers might include:

    a. Pregnancy-induced hypertension.
    b. Inadequate nutrition.
    c. STDs.
    d. Illicit drug use, smoking, and alcohol abuse.

5. Poverty is a strong influence and poverty and minority status are frequently linked.

    Adolescents may turn to pregnancy and parent to achieve the adult status they are desperately seeking. Early academic failure and negative attitudes about school are frequent among this group.

Multiple choice

1. b; 2. c; 3. b; 4. d; 5. a

Matching

1. A; 2. A & B; 3. A; 4. A; 5. A; 6. A & B

True and False

1. True.
2. False.

   Children of adolescent may show less attentive behavior and verbal interaction in preschool and during school-age.

3. True.
4. False.

   Adolescent childbearing effects the adolescent, their children, families and society.

5. False.

   The focus of nursing must be care of individual adolescents and their families along with action at the local, regional, and national level.

ANSWERS TO CHAPTER 10

Key terms

1. G; 2. D; 3. B; 4. H; 5. A; 6. F; 7. E;
8. C

Short answers

1. Possible answers might include:

   a. Past infertility problems.
   b. Increased risk of spontaneous abortion.
   c. Increased incidence of chromosomal abnormalities.
   d. Increased incidence of preexisting medical diseases.
   e. Greater chance of multiple gestation.
   f. Increased risk of preterm labor.
   g. Greater chance of dysfunctional labor, placental problems and cesarean birth.

ANSWERS TO CHAPTER 10

2. Possible answers might include:
   a. Societal pressures.
   b. Motherhood viewed as an essential aspect of married life.
   c. Willingness to establish a stable relationship and complete career training or professional goals.
   d. Economic considerations or achievement of financial security.
   e. Last egg in the basket syndrome.

3. Possible answers might include:
   a. Preconception counseling.
   b. Infertility treatment.
   c. Prenatal and parent education.
   d. Postnatal support groups for older first-time parents.
   e. Individualized care.

Multiple choice

1. b;   2. c;   3. c;   4. d

True and False

1. True.
2. False.

   It is more frequently unplanned.

3. False.

   About 1/3 of women who defer pregnancy after age 35 do so because of an infertility problem.

4. True.
5. True.
6. True.
7. False.

   They may feel more secure which helps achieve paternal role.

8. True.

ANSWERS TO CHAPTER 11

Key terms

1. I;   2. F;   3. J;   4. P;   5. T;   6. C;   7. A;
8. K;   9. D;   10. Q;   11. M;   12. R;   13. .U;   14. S;
15. E;   16. G;   17. V;   18. L;   19. 0;   20. B;   21. N;
22. H

Short answers

1.
   a. Uterus expands, increasing 20-fold in weight; assumes a longitudinal position, displacing intestines. Painless uterine contractions called Braxton Hicks contractions begin about the sixth week.
   b. Breasts become enlarged and sensitive. Nipples become larger, darker, more erectile and areola darkens.
   c. Normal skin variations can include: (1) Chloasma-brown facial pigmentation, (2) Linea nigra-dark vertical abdominal line, (3) Striae-stretch marks in area such as the abdomen, breasts, buttocks and thigh, (4) Spider angiomas-vascular spiders on the chest, (5) Palmer erythema-redness of the palms, (6) Darker pigmentation of nipples, areola, vulva and thighs.
   d. Vaginal and cervical secretions become thickened, white, and acidic.
   e. Gastrointestinal variations may include increased incidence of constipation, heartburn, hemorrhoids, varicosities, nausea, and ptyalism.

2.
   a. Heart appears larger, is pushed upward and to the left; the apex is moved laterally.
   b. Blood volume increases by 50% at the end of the second trimester. Hypervolemia of pregnancy results in a drop in hematocrit to 37% and hemoglobin to 11%.
   c. Cardia output increases 30% to 50% in the first trimester and remains 30% above normal from 30 weeks to term.
   d. Resting heart rate increases to about 78 beats/minute the first trimester, to 85 beats/minute at term.
   e. Stroke volume increases by 30%.
   f. Slight decrease in blood pressure is normal.

Multiple choice

1. h;   2. c;   3. b;   4. d

ANSWERS TO CHAPTER 12

Matching

1. H;   2. I;   3. E;   4. A;   5. G;   6. F;   7. D;
8. C

ANSWERS TO CHAPTER 12

Key terms

1. D;   2. F;   3. L;   4. H;   5. B;   6. E;   7. I;
8. K;   9. M;   10. C;   11. J;   12. G;   13. A

Short answers

1.
   a. Chromosomally normal female.
   b. Turner syndrome female.
   c. Chromosomally normal male.
   d. Trisomy 13 male.
   e. Kleinfelter syndrome.
   f. Cri-du-chat syndrome female.
   g. Trisomy 21, Down syndrome female.

2. Possible answers might include:
   a. Maternal use of over-the-counter drugs.
   b. Alcoholic or drug abusive mother.
   c. Maternal narcotic use, cigarette smoking, and inadequate prenatal nutrition.
   d. Increased maternal age.
   e. Partner is a blood relative.
   f. Particular cultural or race orientation.
   g. Recurrence of disorder in ancestors.
   h. Exposures to teratogenic substances.

3. Possible answers might include:

   a. The lungs do not function as respiratory organs.
   b. Gas exchange function is wholly carried out by the placenta.
   c. Blood flow is for nutrition and excretion purposes only.
   d. Oxygenated blood flows through veins.
   e. Oxygenated and deoxygenated blood passes through the foramen ovale.
   f. Umbilical arteries carry deoxygenated blood back to the placenta.
   g. Small portion of fetal blood circulates to lungs.

4.
   a. Disorders that are clinically expressed when one gene at a given site on an autosomal chromosome is mutant.
   b. Disorders that are clinically expressed when both genes at a given location are mutant.
   c. Disorders determined by genes located on the X chromosome that will be clinically expressed.
   d. Disorders determined by genes located on the X chromosome that may or may not be clinically expressed.

5. Teratogens are agents that cause abnormalities in fetal development. Prenatal exposure to teratogens may cause abortion, intrauterine fetal death, or permanent anatomic, functional, or behavioral abnormalities in the neonate. Teratogens are classified as chemical agents, maternal conditions, or infectious agents.

Multiple choice

1. b; 2. b; 3. d; 4. d; 5. a; 6. c; 7. b;
8. c.

Matching

1. G; 2. E; 3. H; 4. B; 5. F; 6. A; 7. D;
8. I; 9. C

1. A; 2. B; 3. A; 4. C; 5. A; 6. B; 7. A;
8. C; 9. B; 10. B

ANSWERS TO CHAPTER 13

Key terms

1. D; 2. H; 3. F; 4. L; 5. A; 6. I; 7. B;
8. G; 9. J; 10. E; 11. K; 12. C

ANSWERS TO CHAPTER 13

Short Answers

1.

Presumptive Signs	Probable Signs	Positive Signs
Amenorrhea	Abdominal enlargement	Fetal heart tone
Breast tenderness	Ballottement	Fetal movement felt by examiner
Colostrum	Braxton-Hicks Contractions	Ultrasound of fetus
Fatigue	Chadwick's sign	
Morning sickness	Hegar's sign	
Urinary frequency	Quickening	
	Uterine changes	

2. October 22

3. 6-2-0-3-2-0

4. Possible answers might include
   a. Over 35 years old
   b. 3 previous spontaneous abortions
   c. Incompetent cervix
   d. Gestational diabetic
   e. Over weight
   f. Smokes cigarettes

5. Possible answers might include
   a. Health History
   b. Psychosocial Assessment
   c. Physical Examination
   d. Laboratory Tests
   e. Pelvic Examination
   f. Scheduling a return visit

6.

BP: Measured early in pregnancy for a baseline for later comparison. An elevation could indicate development of pregnancy induced hypertension or preeclampsia.

Wt.: Measured in early pregnancy as a baseline for future comparisons of weight loss or gain. Normal weight gain is a minimum of 24 pounds by term. Weight loss could indicate severe nausea and vomiting. Large weight gain may indicate overeating or edema due to preeclampsia

Urine dipstick: Abnormal dipstick results may indicate blood pressure problems, blood sugar problems, poor nutrition, liver or gallbladder disease, urinary tract infection.

7.

12 weeks gestation: The fundus is just rising out of the pelvis. Fetal movement can be detected by ultrasound. At 10-12 weeks fetal heart beat can be heard with a doppler.

16 weeks gestation: The fundus is half-way between the symphysis pubs and umbilicus.

20 weeks gestation: Halfway through the pregnancy. Fundus is at the umbilicus. Fetal movement or quickening has occurred. Fetal heart beat heard with a fetoscope at 18-20 weeks gestation.

8. There is a typical rate of growth for all fetuses. If the above parameters agree with the week gestation as calculated by the EDC, the EDC is reconfirmed. Deviation from findings are indications for further assessments.

9.

First Maneuver: Determines what is in the fundus. Head is hard, smooth, globular, mobile, and ballottable. Breech is soft, irregular, round, and less mobile.

Second Maneuver: Locates the back. Back will feel firm, smooth, convex, and resistant. Small parts will feel small, irregularly placed, and knobby.

Third Maneuver: Identifies the presenting part. Head will feel hard, smooth, and mobile if not engaged. Breech will feel soft and irregular.

Fourth Maneuver: Locates the cephalic prominence. This maneuver may cause discomfort to the woman and may be deferred. Try to determine if the head is flexed.

10. The usual schedule of visits follows:

Every 4 weeks until 28 weeks of pregnancy

Every 2 weeks until 36 weeks of pregnancy.

If problems occur at any time, the visits will become more frequent

Every week until delivery

Multiple choice

1. d;   2. a;   3. c;   4. b;   5. d;   6. a

ANSWERS TO CHAPTER 14

True and False

1. True.
2. False.

    The weeks are 1 to 13; 14-27 and 28 to 40.

3. True
4. False.

    Hbg below 10.5g/100mL or an Hct below 32% indicates anemia.

5. True
6. True
7. True
8. True
9. True
10. False.

    Prenatal assessment by the nurse provides baseline data that are valuable in health maintenance during pregnancy and can contribute to a successful outcome.

ANSWERS TO CHAPTER 14

Key terms

1. J;   2. E;   3. F;   4. B;   5. G;   6. H;   7. L;
8. A;   9. M;   10. D;   11. I;   12. N;   13. C;   14. K

Short answers

1. Possible answers might include:

   a. Uterus measuring large for dates.
   b. Uterus measuring small for dates.
   c. Uncertain LMP.
   d. In order to schedule a procedure such as amniocentesis, chorionic villus sampling, repeat c-section.
   e. Lack of uterine growth.
   f. Absence of FHR or quickening at expected time by history.

2. A full bladder elevates the uterus out of the pelvis so it can be scanned more easily; it also serves as an easily identified landmark. With amniocentesis ultrasound is used to aid in identification of fluid pockets, fetus and placenta. The bladder is empty so it is not inadvertently punctured during the procedure.

3.

Parameters	Nonstress Test	Contraction Stress Test
Description of test	a. Observation of FHR in response to fetal movement.	k. Observing FHR response to induced contractions.
Environment	b. Hospital or doctor's office.	l. Hospital, usually labor and delivery unit.
Client position	c. Sitting, reclining, or supine.	m. Supine.
Length of test	d. 40 minutes needed to determine results.	n. 30 minute baseline strip, then until 3 contractions in 10 minutes are achieved.
Intravenous use	e. No.	o. Yes.
BP evaluation	f. Not needed.	p. Usually every 15 minutes.
Medication used	g. None.	q. Oxytocin.
Monitored parameters	h. Fetal activity; FHR.	r. Contractions; FHR.
Test interpretation	i. A satisfactory test shows FHR accelerations with fetal activity.	s. A satisfactory test shows no late decelerations.
Risk/cost	j. No risk/varies.	t. May stimulate labor/varies.

ANSWERS TO CHAPTER 15   257

4. Amniocentesis is a relatively simple procedure. Mrs. Bolton will be asked to empty her bladder; bare her abdomen, and lie on the bed. FHTs will be monitored before and after the procedure. The ultrasound will be used to locate the fetus, the placenta, and a pocket of fluid. A local anesthetic will be injected into Mrs. Bolton's abdomen. A long needle will be inserted through the abdomen, through the uterus, and into the identified pocket of fluid. About 10 to 20 ml of amniotic fluid will be withdrawn. Gentle pressure will be applied to the puncture site. Mrs. Bolton will be assessed and FHTs monitored for about 30 minutes after which she will be able to go home.

5. Rh sensitivity; extra, broken, or missing chromosomes; damage caused by LSD or other drugs; diseases connected with metabolism or body chemistry; sex of fetus; percentage of chances of sex- linked defects; hemophilia or muscular dystrophy gene.

6. Mrs. Bolton's advanced age. There are greater chances for genetic defects when the mother is older (exp. downs).

7. Amniocentesis is usually performed between the 14th and 17th weeks of gestation because sufficient amniotic fluid is formed by then.

Multiple choice

1. d;   2. a;   3. b;   4. d;   5. d;   6. b;   7. c;
8. b

Matching

1. A, B;   2. A, B, C, D;   3. A, B, C, D, E, F

ANSWERS TO CHAPTER 15

Key terms

1. G;   2. E;   3. C;   4. I;   5. D;   6. F;   7. B;
8. A;   9. H

Short answer

1. Possible answers might include

   a. Age related concerns (adolescent versus over 35)

   b. Social and marital issues/concerns. (Marital status, blended families, lesbian families, etc.).

   c. Previous obstetric history (previous stillbirth, loss, prematurity, C-section, other gynecological problems/surgery)

   d. Psychosocial risk factors (Women with chronic or debilitating illnesses, women without social support).

2. Level of understanding.

3. Immediate concerns.

4. Possible answers might include

    a. Pelvic tilt
    b. Kegels
    c. Walking
    d. Swimming
    e. Aerobic exercises
    f. Stationary biking

ANSWERS TO CHAPTER 15

5.

Minor Discomforts	Description/Cause	Prevention/Nursing Care
Frequent Urination	a. Reduction in bladder capacity due to enlarging uterus.	b. Assess for signs and symptoms of UTI. Normal during 1st and 3rd trimester.
Nausea	c. Related to increased level of progesterone, HCG, and decreased gastric secretions.	d. Usually decreases after 1st trimester. Eat high protein snack at bedtime. Eat crackers before arising. Eat smaller, more frequent meals.
Heartburn	e. Progesterone relaxes the cardiac sphincter, allowing gastric reflux. Enlarging uterus displaces the stomach and duodenum.	f. Most frequent in 3rd trimester. Avoid aggravating foods. Eat frequent small meals. Avoid lying down after eating.
Fatigue	g. Increased demands of cardiopulmonary system, increased metabolic rate. Release of relaxin hormone.	h. Assess fatigue. Normal and temporary during pregnancy. Regular exercise and frequent rest periods encouraged.
Backache	i. Result of lordosis and muscle strain related to the enlarging uterus.	j. Wear low heeled shoes. Exercise regularly, do no heavy lifting, apply local heat, use pelvic tilt exercise.
Headaches	k. Increased circulatory blood volume and heart rate which causes dilation and distension of cerebral arteries.	l. Evaluate headaches. Benign in early pregnancy. Avoid Asprin, rest, relaxation exercises, eat regular meals.
Varicose Veins	m. Cogential weakness in vascular walls; increased blood volume and pressure from enlarging uterus. May be found in legs, vulva, or anal region.	n. Wear supporting stockings, elevate lower extremities, avoid constrictive clothing. Avoid crossing legs. Ambulate frequently. Wear low heeled shoes. Exercise regularly.
Leg Cramps	o. Disturbance in calcium/phosphorus ration; fatigue or muscle strain.	p. Assess. May need to increase dairy products in diet. Keep legs warm, apply local heat, dorsiflex foot.
Edema	q. Normal dependent edema related to sodium and water retention. Increased venous pressure and decreased venous return from legs.	r. Rest in lateral position. Elevate feet. Provide for adequate protein intake, consume ample fluids, use normal salt intake.
Vaginal Discharge	s. Increase normal due to increased cervical mucous caused by estrogen and increased vascularity.	t. Avoid panty hose. Wear loose cotton underwear. Avoid tight pants. Keep perineum clean and dry.

6. Possible danger signs and symptoms might include:

    a. Any sudden onset of frank, profuse vaginal bleeding can be a sign of ectopic pregnancy or threatened abortion placenta previa, or abruptio placentae.
    b. Dizziness associated with pelvic or uterine pain can indicate ectopic pregnancy or abruptio placentae with hidden bleeding.
    c. Rhythmic tightening (contracting) of the uterus. Constant low abdominal cramping or low back pain. Could be premature labor or urinary track infection.
    d. Sudden gush of fluid from the vagina. Indicates rupture of membranes/preterm labor.
    e. Generalized edema, especially of face and hands. Indicates pregnancy-induced hypertension, or toxemia.
    f. Rapid weight gain over several days. Indicated pregnancy-induced hypertension.
    g. Flashing lights, spots before eyes, or double vision. Associated with pregnancy-incuded hypertension.
    h. Vomiting that will not go away. Leads to dehydration.
    i. Decrease or absence of fetal activity. Sign of fetal distress or demise.

7. Possible answers might include:

    a. Repeated accidents.
    b. Depression.
    c. Alcohol or drug use.
    d. Missed appointments with healing injuries present.
    e. Any head, neck, abdomen, genital, or breast injury.
    f. Cigarette burns.
    g. Trauma to the face.
    h. Mulitple injuries at different healing phases.

Multiple choice

1. c;   2. c;   3. b;   4. d;   5. b;   6. b;   7. c;
8. c;   9. d;   10. b

True and False

1. True.
2. False.

    The needs should be identified by the client/family.

3. True.
4. True.
5. False.

The nurse must interview the woman in a supportive, nonthreatening way in a setting the ensures privacy.

ANSWERS TO CHAPTER 16

Key terms

1. G; 2. C; 3. J; 4. P; 5. K; 6. H; 7. L;
8. B; 9. M; 10. U; 11. N; 12. A; 13. I; 14. O;
15. R; 16. D; 17. F; 18. T; 19. Q; 20. S; 21. E

Short answers

1.
   a. Rh incompatibility
   b. Indirect Coombs' test
   c. 28

2. Painless vaginal bleeding.

3. Possible answers might include:
   a. Nausea and vomiting occurring in first 16 weeks.
   b. Accompanied by disturbances of appetite.
   c. Causes alterations in nutritional status such as; weight loss, electrolyte imbalance, and ketosis with ketonuria.
   d. Is intractable in nature.

4. The ability of the cervix to maintain a pregnancy to term because of a structural or functional defect.

5.
   a. Watchful waiting.
   b. Placement of a cervical cerclage.

6. Jonie is not a candidate for RhoGAM because her indirect Coombs' test indicates that she has already been sensitized to Rh+ blood and has developed antibodies. Because the first baby was Rh- there is no way to know when Jonie became sensitized. it could be possible that she had an undiagnosed miscarriage between the two pregnancies. She could have received a blood transfusion or have had a small placental bleed during this pregnancy. It

is important for Jonie to receive a clear explanation of the risks she faces for hemolytic disease in future pregnancies. Jonie's newborn needs to be evaluated carefully.

7. 6 g/dL.

8. Slight enlargement of the kidneys.

    Dilation of renal pelves and ureters

    Elongation of the ureters.

    Changes in bladder position.

    Changes in urine composition, such as glucosuria, which support bacterial growth.

9.
    a. Extreme irritability and agitation.
    b. Hypertonicity.
    c. Diarrhea.
    d. Dehydration.

10. Abruptio placentae.

Multiple choice

1. b;   2. c;   3. d;   4. a;   5. d;   6. b;   7. b;
8. c;   9. b;   10. d

Matching

1. B;   2. E;   3. F;   4. C;   5. H;   6. G;   7. I;
8. A;   9. D

True and False

1. True.
2. False.

    Most require careful ongoing assessment to identify problems and correct them.

3. True.
4. False.

    Because antibiotics cross the placenta, consideration of the fetus must be made when prescribing therapy.

5. True.
6. True.
7. True.

8. True.
9. True.
10. False.

Treatment generally is toward maintaining maternal and fetal physiologic stability.

ANSWERS TO CHAPTER 17

Key terms

1. J;   2. D;   3. E;   4. H;   5. I;   6. B;   7. F;
8. G;   9. A;   10. C

Short answers

1. Possible answers might include:

   a. Being overweight or underweight
   b. Having a short stature
   c. Inadequate or excessive weight gain during pregnancy
   d. Anemia before or during pregnancy
   e. Being hypovolemic
   f. Experiencing an obstetrical complication in previous pregnancy
   g. Being 18 years of age or younger
   h. Being in a low income group
   i. Having a known nutritional deficiency
   j. History of substance abuse during pregnancy
   k. Experiencing pica.

2. Below 12.0 g/dL; below 35 vol%
   Below 10.0 g/dL; below 30.0 vol%
   Below 11.0 gld/; below 33.0 vol%

3. Possible answers might include:

     The client's general health history

     A physical assessment of the client, noting an evidence of nutritional abnormalities.

     A review of lab tests, especially CBC, albumin and cholesterol levels if available.

     A 24 hour diet recall with questions concerning the meaning or value of food and food consumption to the client.

     Socioeconomic status of client and number of persons relying on same source of income.

     Cultural/ethnic group and specific beliefs of that group that may affect nutritional status during pregnancy.

     History or evidence of substance abuse by client.

4. All substances ingested by the mother may affect her health and the health of her unborn infant. Alcohol is not a required nutrient and has no nutritional value; also, it has been linked with the development of specific birth defects in infants of mothers who consumed alcohol during pregnancy. Caffeine is a substance found in many foods, beverages, and drugs. Recommendations are to decrease caffeine ingestion during pregnancy because it may be linked with problems such as skeletal anomalies, and low birth weight.

Multiple choice

1. c;   2. d;   3. b;   4. c;   5. a;   6. d

Matching

1. C;   2. D;   3. I;   4. A;   5. H;   6. B;   7. E;
8. G;   9. F

True and False

1. True.
2. False.

   Increased nutritional requirements.

3. True.
4. False.

   Vitamin and mineral supplementation is not recommended unless the woman is at nutritional risk.

5. True.
6. True.
7. True.
8. True.

ANSWERS TO CHAPTER 18

Key terms

1. D;   2. C;   3. A;   4. B;   5. I;   6. E;   7. J;
8. G;   9. H;   10. F

Short answers

1. Possible answers might include:

   a. Human reproduction including anatomy, physiology, and psychology from conception through postpartum health care.

   b. Nutritional needs and relationship to fetal development.

   c. Self-help techniques and comfort measures.

   d. Role and support techniques for companion.

   e. Social and psychological family roles.

   f. Roles of health care providers.

   g. Options in labor and birth procedures.

   h. Rights of expectant family.

   i. High-risk birth and prenatal testing.

   j. Preparation for parenting.

   k. Tour of maternity-newborn unit.

2.
   a. To provide the childbearing couple with the knowledge and skills they need to cope with the stress of pregnancy, labor, and birth.

   b. To prepare the childbearing couple to become informed consumers of maternity care.

   c. To assist the childbearing couple in achieving a safe, positive, and rewarding birth experience.

3.

(A)	Creating a mental picture and recalling the sensations of a pleasurable or relaxing scene.	vs.	(B)	Focusing attention on an external point, object or sound.
(C)	Systematic tensing and releasing of muscle groups in a pattern which leads to deep relaxation of entire body.	vs.	(D)	The tensing and relaxing of some muscle groups while maintaining deep relaxation elsewhere.
(E)	Rubbing back and shoulders with gentle pressure with lotion or powder.	vs.	(F)	A light, rhythmic, circular stroking of the abdomen with the fingertips.

Multiple choice

1. d; 2. d; 3. c; 4. b; 5. c

Matching

1. C; 2. A; 3. B; 4. E; 5. D; 6. F

True and False

1. True.
2. False.
   These things have become an important nursing priority.
3. True.
4. True.
5. True.

ANSWER TO CHAPTER 19

Key terms

1. R;   2. E;   3. O;   4. H;   5. K;   6. N;   7. P;
8. I;   9. D;   10. L; 11. A; 12. F; 13. S; 14. U;
15. M; 16. Q; 17. G; 18. J; 19. T; 20. C; 21. V;
22. B

Short answers

1.
   a. Passage - The pelvic anatomy must be spacious enough to accommodate the fetus.
   b. Passenger - The fetus must be in an advantageous position and small enough to fit through the passage.
   c. Powers - Uterine contractions must be rhythmic, coordinated, and efficient enough to dilate and efface the cervix.
   d. Psyche - Maternal emotional resources must be adequate to accomplish the delivery of the fetus.

ANSWERS TO CHAPTER 19

2.

	Location	Measurement
Diagnoal Conjugate	a. The distance from the lower margin of the symphysis publis to the promontory of the sacrum	11.5 to 12.0.
Obstetric Conjugate	b. The shortest distance between the promontory of the sacrum and the symphysis pubis	10 cm or more.
Biischial Diameter	c. The distance between the two ischial tuberosities	10 cm or more.

3. Possible answers might include:

   a. Leopold's maneuvers.
   b. Visual inspection of the maternal abdomen.
   c. Location of the fetal heart tones.
   d. Vaginal examination.
   e. Visualization by ultrasound.

4. Sutures

   Fontanelle

5.

	Location	Measurement
Soboccipitobregmatic diameter	a. The smallest diameter of the fetal skull from the lower edge of the occipital bone to the forehead	averages 9.5 cm.
Biparietal diameter	b. The distance between the parietal bosses and represents the largest transverse diameter of the head	averages 9.25 cm.

6.
- a. Frank breech - most common, characterized by flexion of the fetal thighs and extension of the knees; the feet rest alongside the fetal head.
- b. Complete breech - characterized by flexion of the fetal thighs and knees; the fetus appears to be in a squatting position.
- c. Footling or incomplete breech - One or both feet may present through the cervix.

7.

    a. 3;   b. 1;   c. 4;   d. 6;   e. 2;   f. 5

8.
- a. Left occiput anterior
- b. Left occiput posterior
- c. Right sacrum anterior
- d. Right mentum anterior
- e. Left occiput transverse
- f. Right sacrum posterior

   (mother - baby - mother)

9.
- a. Labor begins when the uterus is stretched to a certain point.
- b. The descent of the presenting part stimulates pressure receptors in the lower uterine segment. This causes increased secretion of oxytocin by the maternal posterior pituitary gland. Oxytocin stimulates the myometrium to contract and start labor.
- c. Oxytocin receptor in the uterine muscle increase near the end of gestation. Oxytocin promotes the release of prostaglandin F_2 alpha from the uterine endometrial decidua. As progesterone levels decrease, prostaglandin formation increases. Maturation of fetal adrenal glands and the release of fetal cortisol has been suggested.
- d. The release of bioactive agents from the uterine decidua into amniotic fluid. Platelet - activating factor stimulates the production of prostaglandin E_2 by fetal membranes. Arachidonic acid is a precursor of prostaglandin which stimulates contractions.

10.
- a. First stage of labor - begins with true labor and ends with complete dilatation of the cervix.
- b. Second stage of labor - begins with complete dilatation of the cervix and ends with the birth of the baby.
- c. Third stage of labor - begins with the birth of the baby and ends with the delivery of the placenta.
- d. The fourth stage of labor begins with the delivery of the placenta and lasts for several (approximately 4) hours.

ANSWERS TO CHAPTER 19

11.
- a. Braxton Hicks contractions increase.
- b. Lightening about 2-3 weeks prior to labor.
- c. Cervical and vaginal changes; increased vaginal discharge.
- d. Weight loss and gastrointestinal upset.
- e. Nesting behavior - need to have everything ready.

12.
- a. Uterine contractions that cause the uterus to dilate and efface.
- b. Spontaneous rupture of membranes.
- c. Bloody show - blood-tinged vaginal secretions.

Multiple choice

1. d; 2. b; 3. d; 4. b; 5. a; 6. c; 7. a;
8. c

True and False

1. True
2. False.
   The maneuvers are predictable and synchronized.
3. False.
   In most cases the diameter of the head is the largest.
4. True.
5. True.
6. False.
   Primigravidas may have 14 to 15 hours of labor and multigravidas 8.
7. True.
8. True.
9. False.
   All this happens during the fourth stage.
10. True.

ANSWERS TO CHAPTER 20

Key terms

1. K;   2. J;   3. D;   4. E;   5. B;   6. I;   7. G;
8. C;   9. H;   10. F;   11. A

Short answers

1. Possible answers might include:

    Are your contractions regular?

    Are they getting closer together?

    Have the contractions become any stronger or longer since they began?

    What happens to the contractions when you walk?

    Where are you feeling the contractions?

    Have you had a sudden gush of fluid?

    Have you noticed any bloody-show?

    What relaxation techniques have you used?

2. Cervical dilatation and effacement
   Fetal station.

3.

Status of membranes	Intact, ruptured, or bulging.
Status of Cervix:	Soft, firm, dilatation, and effacement
Fetal presentation:	Presenting part, fetal position
Fetal station:	Relationship of presenting part to ischial spines
Engagement:	Presenting part applied or floating

4. When there is vaginal bleeding.

5. With mild contractions, fingertips can indent the abdomen easily (similar to feeling the fleshy part of the cheeks). With moderate contractions, it feels similar tot he chin (fingers can indent the fundus only slightly). With strong contractions, it feels like the forehead (fingers cannot indent the abdomen).

6. Time contractions in minutes from beginning of one contraction to the beginning of the next.

ANSWERS TO CHAPTER 20

7. Time duration in seconds from beginning to end of a contraction.

8.
    a. Time of rupture
    b. Color of fluid
    c. Odor of fluid (if any)
    d. Consistency of fluid
    e. FHR after rupture

9. Call the health care provider for c, d, f, and g.

10. Latent Phase: A and D.
    Active Phase: E, H, and J.
    Transition: B, C, F, G, and I.

Multiple choice

1. c;   2. b;   3. d;   4. a;   5. d;   6. c;   7. a;
8. b;   9. c;   10. d

Matching

1. F;   2. C;   3. D;   4. A;   5. B;   6. E

True and False

1. False.

   The time is often accompanied by feelings of heightened anticipation, anxiety, and uncertainty.

2. True.
3. True.
4. True.
5. False.

   The goals include assistance with comfort measures and pain control efforts, assumption of self-care activities, and continued encouragement of the support person.

6. True.
7. True.
8. False.

   Close collaboration with the coach is essential.

ANSWERS TO CHAPTER 21

Key terms

1. D; 2. B; 3. F; 4. H; 5. C; 6. E; 7. A;
8. G

Short answers

1.
   a. Uterine contractions
   b. Bearing-down efforts of the mother.

2. Exertion of labor causes the woman to become warm. Mouth-breathing with bearing-down efforts cause mouth dryness; as does dehydration. The frozen bars and lollipops provide a small amount of energy and change the taste in the clients mouth.

3. Teach Teri open-glottis or gentle pushing. Ask her to push in short, 6 to 7 second periods and only when she has the urge to do so (not continuously through each contraction). The urge to push comes 3 to 5 times during each contraction. Tell Terri to exhale slightly as she pushes. It is okay if she makes grunting or other expiratory sounds.

4. Possible answers might include:

   a. The position should facilitate physiologic labor and birth.
   b. The position should allow bearing-down efforts to be aided by gravity.
   c. The position should promote fetal descent and rotation by providing for mobility of the pelvis into a pelvic tilt, creating larger pelvic diameters.
   d. The position should not cause supine hypotension.
   e. No position is "ideal". Choice of position must be evaluated according to individual circumstances.
   f. Excessive pressure on calf or popliteal area is to be avoided.
   g. The woman must not be left alone, once positioned.
   h. The woman's modesty should be respected.
   i. Perineum should be easily viewed and accessed.

ANSWERS TO CHAPTER 21

5. Possible answers might include:

   a. Apply warm compresses to the perineum during the second stage of labor to promote relaxation, increased circulation, and increased pliability of the perineal tissues.

   b. Encourage gentle pushing during the second stage to allow for gradual distention of the perineal tissue.

   c. Encourage the patient to avoid bearing-down efforts when crowning occurs.

   d. Use a lubricant to massage the perineum during the second stage.

   e. Apply an icepack on the clitoral or periurethral area during crowning to reduce the burning and stinging that accompany stretching of the vagina, and to enhance perineal relaxation.

   f. Use maternal positions for delivery that avoid overstretching the perineum, such as the sidelying or semisitting positions. When stirrups are used, position to avoid hyperextension of the legs and extreme perineal stretching.

6. To help in controlling the birth and to reduce the risk of an over-rapid delivery. The head is usually delivered between contractions.

7. Nuchal cord is a loop of umbilical cord around the baby's neck.

8.
   a. Slight gush of blood from the vagina.

   b. Lengthening of the cord.

   c. Rising, rounded uterine fundus palpable through the abdomen.

9.

	Baby A	Baby B	Baby C	Baby D	Baby E
Heart Rate	2	0	1	2	2
Respiratory Rate	1	1	2	2	2
Muscle tone	1	0	2	1	2
Refex irritability	1	1	2	0	2
Color	1	0	1	1	2
Totals	6	2	8	6	10

10. Possible answers might include:

   a. Suctioning nasopharynx with bulb syringe.

   b. Deep suctioning with mechanical suction device.

   c. Positioning to facilitate drainage of secretions on abdomen, head turned to side.

11. With one hand anchor the lower uterine segment just above the symphysis pubis; with the other, gently massage the fundal area. Massage gently, with adequate support of the lower segment. Do only when fundus is not firm.

12. Massage stimulates the myometrium to contract, promoting hemostasis and expulsion of clots. Over stimulation can contribute to muscle fatigue and a tendency toward relaxation.

13. The uterine suspensory ligaments are relaxed after delivery and offer little resistance. Aggressive massage may result in uterine prolapse.

14.
    a. Uterine atony
    b. Retained placental fragments.

15. A fever in the first 24 hours post delivery, in the absence of premature rupture of membranes, is most likely due to dehydration. You should replace Sharon's fluids, either orally or by I.V.

16.
    1. N; 2. A; 3. A; 4. N; 5. N; 6. N;
    7. A; 8. A

17. Possible answers might include:
    a. Progressing from tentative touching to confident touching and enfolding.
    b. Active reaching for infant.
    c. Active attempts to make and hold eye contact (enface).
    d. Expressions of approval or satisfaction with infant's sex, weight, appearance, and size.

18.
    a. Neonatal respiratory problems.
    b. Hypothermia.
    c. Hypoglycemia.

Multiple choice

1. c; 2. b; 3. d; 4. c; 5. d; 6. c; 7. a;
8. c; 9. d; 10. c

ANSWERS TO CHAPTER 22

Matching

Lacerations

1. F;   2. E;   3. A;   4. B;   5. C;   6. D

Thermoregulation

1. C;   2. A;   3. B;   4. C;   5. C (possible A and B); 6. B (possibly C)

True and False

1. False.

    Characterized by a decrease.

2. True.
3. True.
4. True.
5. False.

    The nurse remains at the woman's side, offering final words of encouragement and remaining ready to assist the birth attendant.

6. True.
7. False.

    Many women experience a sudden surge of energy and fatigue and pain is temporarily forgotten.

8. True.
9. True.

ANSWERS TO CHAPTER 22

Key terms

1. A;   2. H;   3. C;   4. B;   5. G;   6. E;   7. I;
8. J;   9. F;   10. D

276 STUDY GUIDE TO ACCOMPANY MATERNAL AND NEONATAL NURSING

Short answers

1.
   a. E, no evident FHR problem.
   b. I, tachycardia, poor beat-to-beat variability.
   c. I, minimal long-term variability.
   d. E, no evident FHR problems (but observe since has early decelerations; accelerations are desirable).
   e. I, variable decelerations.

2.

Type	Cause	Characteristics	Clinical Significance
Early deceleration	Vagal stimulation from head compression	Mirror image of contraction	Usually innocuous
Late deceleration	Uteroplacental insufficiency	Onset at peak of contraction	ends after contraction
Variable deceleration	Umbilical cord compression	Decelerations unrelated to contractions	Possible severe fetal compromise

3.
   a. Turn the woman to the left or right side.
   b. Discontinue oxytocin infusion if going.
   c. Administer oxygen by face mask at 8 to 12L/min.
   d. Start or increase IV fluids.
   e. Reassure and support the woman.
   f. Prepare for possible intrauterine amnioinfusion or emergency delivery.

Multiple choice

1. a;   2. d;   3. a;   4. c;   5. c

ANSWERS TO CHAPTER 23   277

True and False

1. True.
2. False.

   The nurse collaborates with the birth attendant and provides the woman with information and emotional support.

3. True.
4. False.

   The heart rate should accelerate.

5. True.

ANSWERS TO CHAPTER 23

Key terms

1. C;   2. O;   3. L;   4. P;   5. G;   6. B;   7. Q;
8. R;   9. A;   10. F;   11. H;   12. D;   13. I;   14. N;
15. M;   16. E;   17. J;   18. K

Short answers

1. Placental insufficiency is associated with postterm pregnancy.

2. The amniotic sac is punctured during a vaginal exam. This is a painless procedures; however, she will experience warm and wet sensations from the amniotic fluid.

3.
   a. Assemble equipment (amnihook, sterile gloves, lubricant, linens, Doptone).
   b. Position the patient on her back with her knees flexed and apart.
   c. Monitor fetal heart tones.

4.
   a. Assess fetal heart tones.
   b. Assess the color, amount, and odor of amniotic fluid.
   c. Explain to the woman what to expect now that the membranes are ruptured.
   d. Change bed linens as needed.
   e. Assess maternal temperature every 2 hours.

5.
   a. Assess uterine activity every 15 minutes, including manual palpation of fundus.
   b. Assess fetal heart tones every 15 minutes.
   c. Assess maternal vital signs every 15 minutes.
   d. Assess intake and output.
   e. Assess maternal pain and fatigue.

6. Assess what they understand about the situation and offer information. Explain sequence of events for the delivery. Give the couple rationale for performing certain procedures (prep, foley catheter) and explain post-recovery routine (if time allows).

7. Support the family's coping mechanisms. Promote maternal comfort. Encourage father's presence to support Sue during preparation and in delivery room. Allow couple time to see and/or hold newborn as soon as possible.

8. Skin cut is transverse at the level of mons pubis. A horizontal incision is made in the lower segment of the uterus.

9. Yes, as long as she chooses a birth facility with availability for emergency surgery. She meets other criteria, because this was her first pregnancy, with the low-segment cesarean performed for fetal distress.

10. Outlet forceps application are done when the fetal head is visible at the vaginal introitus without separating the labia. The forceps are curved metal tongs used to facilitate the birth of the infants head by providing traction and rotation.

Multiple choice

1. a;   2. b;   3. d;   4. c;   5. b

True and False

1. False.

   The nurse plays a central role.

2. True.

3. False.

   The nurse plays an important role in the procedure.

4. True.

ANSWERS TO CHAPTER 24

Key terms

1. C;   2. A;   3. E;   4. D;   5. B

Short answers

1. It decreases the amount of medication transferred to the fetus, since placental circulation is markedly decreased during uterine contractions.

2. Maternal hypotension and/or respiratory depression.

3. Nausea.

4. Left side-lying.

5. The anesthesia decreases bladder sensation.

6. Transient fetal bradycardia.

7. Hydration with 500-1000 cc IV fluid.

8. Maintain bed rest and hydrate adequately.

9. They rapidly cross the placenta to the fetus and cause varying depths of CNS depression.

10. Vomiting, aspiration, and postpartum hemorrhage.

Multiple choice

1. a;   2. b;   3. c;   4. d;   5. c

Matching

1. D;   2. E;   3. A;   4. C;   5. B

True and False

1. True.
2. False.
   The nurse must monitor both maternal and fetal well-being.
3. True.

4. False.

The significant other becomes the link between mother and infant until the mother resumes consciousness.

5. True.

ANSWERS TO CHAPTER 25

Key terms

1. C;   2. D;   3. A;   4. E;   5. G;   6. F;   7. B

Short answers

1.
   a. Perceptions of the event.
   b. Situational support.
   c. Coping mechanisms.

2.
   a. Shock.
   b. Denial and disbelief.
   c. Anger.
   d. Sadness and guilt.
   e. Reorganization and resolution.

3. Bed rest at home or in the hospital.

4.
   a. Loneliness.
   b. Boredom.
   c. Powerlessness.
   d. Loss of control.

Multiple choice

1. b;   2. c;   3. c

ANSWERS TO CHAPTER 26

True and False

1. True.
2. False.

   Behavioral and verbal clues assist nurses to initiate appropriate nursing interventions.

3. True.

ANSWERS TO CHAPTER 26

Key terms

1. D;   2. L;   3. E;   4. N;   5. C;   6. F;   7. G;
8. I;   9. J;   10. M;   11. A;   12. K;   13. O;   14. B;
15. H.

Short answers

1. Possible answers might include:

   a. Preterm labor.
   b. Preeclampsia.
   c. Third trimester bleeding.
   d. Maternal diseases (diabetes, hypertension).
   e. Rh sensitization.
   f. Drug abuse
   g. Multiple gestation.

2.
   a. Ascending infections from the vagina across intact or through ruptured membranes.
   b. Transplacental infection from the maternal circulation to the amniotic sac.
   c. Descending infection from the abdominal cavity through the fallopian tubes and into the uterus.

3.
   a. Upper gastrointestinal abnormalities.
   b. Anencephaly.
   c. Hydrops fetalis.
   d. Hydrocephalus.
   e. Neural tube defects.

4. Possible answers might include:

    a. Abnormal fetal position: breech, shoulder, face, or brow.
    b. Multifetal gestation.
    c. Prematurity.
    d. Polyhydramnios.
    e. Fetopelvic disproportion.
    f. Abnormally long umbilical cord.
    g. Rupture of membranes before engagement of the presenting part.

5. Cesarean delivery. Because of the potential for hypotonic uterine contractions; fetal complications; and malpresentation of one or both fetuses.

6.
    a. Nonreactive nonstress test.
    b. Sudden decrease in total volume of amniotic fluid.
    c. Amniotic fluid volume index of 5 cm or less.
    d. Decreasing biophysical profile score.
    e. Evidence of placental aging, determined by ultrasound grading of the placenta.

7.
    a. Fetal size, presentation, position, and ability of the fetal head to mold in the pelvis.
    b. Ability of the uterus to contract efficiently.
    c. Pelvic size and internal shape.
    d. Structural abnormalities.

8. Because the buttocks are soft and are not as effective as the head in dilating the cervix. The head may become entrapped after the body is delivered and fetal hypoxia and asphyxia may occur.

9. When the total length of labor is 3 hours or less, the diagnosis of precipitous labor is confirmed.

10. Uterine Rupture.

11.
    a. Septic shock.
    b. Placental or profuse uterine bleeding.
    c. Release of fetal thromboplastin and eclampsia.

12. Amniotic fluid embolism.

ANSWERS TO CHAPTER 27

Multiple choice

1. c;   2. a;   3. a;   4. c;   5. b;   6. c;   7. d;
8. c

Matching

1. A;   2. B;   3. A;   4. B;   5. A;   6. B;   7. B

True and False

1. True.
2. False.
   "Medical diagnosis alone" should be changed to "The nursing process".
3. True.
4. True.
5. False.
   Maternal well-being also is threatened.
6. True.
7. False.
   Maternal well-being is important but the nurse in this case needs to focus on fetal well-being.
8. True.
9. True.
10. True.

ANSWERS TO CHAPTER 27

Key terms

1. I;   2. F;   3. G;   4. C;   5. A;   6. M;   7. D;
8. L;   9. H;   10. E;   11. K;   12. J;   13. B

Short answers

1. Possible answers might include:
   a. Polyhydramnios.
   b. Prenatal bleeding.
   c. Multifetal gestation.
   d. Prior preterm delivery.
   e. Cervical incompetence.
   f. Uterine or cervical anomalies.
   g. Reproductive tact infection.
   h. Poor pregnancy weight gain.
   i. Abdominal surgery during pregnancy.
   j. Previous second trimester abortion.
   k. Cervical dilatation more than 2 cm by 32 weeks.

2. The diagnosis of preterm labor is based on the presence of uterine contractions and the finding of progressive cervical effacement or dilatation.

3. Bed rest and hydration.

4. Nervousness, restlessness, tremors, headache, insomnia, hypertension, tachycardia, and palpitations.

5.
   a. Size of fetus.
   b. Position of Fetus.
   c. Presence of infection.
   d. Presence of cord prolapse.

6.
   a. TPR hourly.
   b. Limited vaginal exams.
   c. Assess odor, color, amount of fluid.
   d. Maintain bed rest if fetal head is not engaged.
   e. Monitor fetal heart rate.

ANSWERS TO CHAPTER 27

7. Possible answers might include:

   a. First pregnancy or first pregnancy with current partner.

   b. Nullipara under age 21 and multipara over age 35.

   c. Family prevalence of PIH.

   d. Preexisting diabetes or renal disease.

   e. Preexisting chronic hypertension.

   f. Multifetal pregnancy.

   g. Hydatidiform mole.

   h. Hydrops fetalis.

8.
   a. Hypertension.

   b. Edema.

   c. Proteinuria.

9. Tonoclonic seizures.

10. H: Hemolysis of red blood cells.

    EL: Elevated liver enzymes.

    LP: Low platelet count (less than 100,000).

11. Vaginal and urinary tract infection; pregnancy-induced hypertension; fetal malformations; polyhydramnios; macrosomia; sudden fetal death near term; prematurity; respiratory distress with early delivery; birth injury from macrosomia.

12.
    a. Serum or urine estriol determinations.

    b. Nonstress testing or contraction stress testing.

    c. Ultrasonography.

    d. HPL and PG via amniocentesis.

13.
    a. A slow onset of congestive heart failure.

    b. An acute episode of heart failure with pulmonary edema.

14.
    a. V.S. every 15 minutes; report to doctor if respiratory rate is above 24/min., or if pulse rate is above 100.

    b. Continuous electronic monitoring.

    c. Positioned in left lateral recumbent position.

    d. Bearing down efforts should be avoided.

Multiple choice

1. b; 2. a; 3. d; 4. d; 5. a; 6. d; 7. c;
8. a; 9. d; 10. c

True and False

1. False.

   It tends to increase heart rate.

2. True.
3. True.
4. True.
5. True.

ANSWERS TO CHAPTER 28

Key terms

1. E; 2. L; 3. F; 4. B; 5. G; 6. H; 7. J;
8. I; 9. C; 10. D; 11. A; 12. K

Short answers

1. Six.
2. Puerperium.
3. 10-12.
4. Baby, placenta, and amniotic fluid.
5. 400-500 cc, diuresis, and diaphoresis.
6. Estrogen, progesterone, and prolactin.
7. Colostrum.
8. Third.
9. Engorged.
10. Oxytocin, suckling.
11. Involution.

12. Lochia.

13. Placental.

14. After pains.

15.
   a. Midway between umbilicus and symphysis on midline.
   b. One finger breadth (1 cm) above or at the umbilicus.
   c. Three finger breadths (3 cm) below the umbilicus.
   d. Not palpable above the symphysis.

Multiple choice

1. c; 2. d; 3. b; 4. c; 5. c; 6. b; 7. a;
8. d; 9. d; 10. c

True and False

1. True.
2. False.
   Changes are reversed by the fourth to sixth week.
3. True.
4. True.
5. False.
   They do not experience the changes; however, they do have similar needs.
6. True.

ANSWERS TO CHAPTER 29

Key terms

1. C; 2. J; 3. D; 4. H; 5. I; 6. A; 7. G;
8. E; 9. B; 10. F; 11. K; 12. N; 13. L; 14. M

Short answers

1. Possible answers might include:

   a. Grand multiparity (five or more births).
   b. Previous history of uterine atony.
   c. Over distension of the uterus due to polyhydramnios, a large fetus, or multiple gestation.
   d. Presence of uterine fibroids.
   e. Chorioamnionitis during labor.
   f. Precipitous labor and delivery.
   g. Prolonged first or second stage of labor (or both).
   h. Oxytocin induction or augmentation of labor.
   i. Magnesium sulfate infusion during labor and delivery.
   j. Use of general anesthesia.
   k. Full bladder after delivery.

2.
   a. Involving the skin or vaginal mucosa but not extending into muscular layers.
   b. Extending from the skin and vaginal mucosa into the muscles of the perineum.
   c. Extending from the skin, vaginal mucosa, and muscle into the anal sphincter.
   d. Extending through the rectal mucosa into the lumen of the rectum.

3. Possible answers might include:

   a. Bearing-down efforts after delivery.
   b. Precipitous delivery with woman in standing position.
   c. Traction on the umbilical cord before placental separation.
   d. Vigorous kneading of the fundus to cause placental separation and expulsion.
   e. Excessive manual pressure on the fundus.
   f. Delivery of a neonate with a short cord.
   g. Manual extraction of placenta.
   h. Rapid delivery with multiple gestation.

ANSWERS TO CHAPTER 29

4. Possible answers might include:
   a. Wipe from front to back after voiding or defecating.
   b. Clean perineum after each void or defecation with squirt bottle.
   c. Change perineal pads frequently.
   d. Encourage sitz bath.
   e. Encourage forcing fluids and voiding frequently.
   f. Teach proper breast care and breastfeeding techniques.
   g. Use strict asepsis with IVs.

5.
   a. Positive Homans' sign.
   b. Swelling in the affective leg.
   c. Muscle pain in the affected leg.
   d. Tenderness to touch in the affected leg.
   e. Induration along the vein in the affected leg.

Multiple choice

1. d;   2. b;   3. b;   4. b;   5. c;   6. d;   7. b;
8. c;   9. a;   10. c

Matching

1. A;   2. C;   3. B;   4. D

True and False

1. False.
   Cesarean section increases both maternal morbidity and mortality.

2. False.
   Fundal tone, pulse, and blood pressure are most important indicators of postpartum hemorrhage.

3. True.
4. False.
   Abruptio placenta causes afibrinogenemia which contributes to postpartum hemorrhage.

5. True.
6. True.

7. False.

Costovertebral angle tenderness is a sign of kidney infection (pyelonephritis).

8. True.

ANSWERS TO CHAPTER 30

Key terms

1. F; 2. K; 3. M; 4. T; 5. G; 6. O; 7. X;
8. Y; 9. H; 10. C; 11. L; 12. E; 13. N; 14. C;
15. P; 16. J; 17. B; 18. Q; 19. S; 20. I; 21. W;
22. R; 23. U; 24. A; 25. V

Short answers

1. Surfactant.

2.
    a. Chemical stimuli: Transient asphyxia occurs. Chemoreceptors are stimulated by the lowered arterial oxygen tension, the elevated arterial carbon dioxide tension, and the decrease in arterial pH. Impulses triggered by these chemoreceptors stimulate the respiratory center in the medulla.

    b. Sensory stimuli: Tactile, visual, auditory, and olfactory stimuli contribute to the initiation of respiration.

    c. Thermal stimuli: When the newborn's warm, wet body is delivered, evaporation causes an immediate drop in the skin temperature. Thermal receptors relay impulses to the medulla triggering the first breath.

    d. Mechanical stimuli: During the passage through the birth canal, approximately 30% of the fetal lung fluid filling the airways and alveoli is squeezed out. With vaginal births, recoil of the chest wall occurs, drawing air into the partially cleared passages.

3.
    a. Closure of the Foramen Ovale.

    b. Closure of the Ductus Arteriosus.

    c. Closure of the Ductus Venosus.

4. Newborns are prone to heat loss because they have a large surface area in relation to their body weight. The newborn responds to cold stress by increasing the metabolic rate. Norepinephrine is released at nerve endings in brown fat. There is an increased demand for oxygen and glucose. With prolonged cold stress, brown fat and glucose stores are depleted which can result in hypothermia and hypoglycemia.

5. Liver-synthesized Vitamin K.

ANSWERS TO CHAPTER 30

6. 40 to 60; 90

7. 24 hours; brick-dust; 20.

8. Third to fifth.

9. Immature.

10.
   a. 15-30 minutes; eyes open, vigorous activity including crying, rapid irregular respirations and heart rate; strong sucking reflex.

      Support temperature regulation by drying and placing under warmer; allow parents time for bonding; observe for respiratory instability; maintain airway; encourage nursing if breastfeeding.

   b. 2-4 hours; quieter, sleeping and difficult to rouse; respiratory and heart rates slow to resting/baseline level; temperature drops; bowel sounds become audible.

      Observe for transition signs; monitor VS; position to facilitate drainage of respiratory secretions; obtain blood glucose per agency policy; maintain neutral thermal environment; offer fluids per agency policy/physician's order.

   c. 4-6 hours; respiratory and heart rate change rapidly; periods of tachypnea, gagging, regurgitation of mucus; transient cyanosis alternates with periods of quiet sleep; bowel sounds increase; increased interest in eating.

      Observe VS; maintain neutral thermal environment; position to facilitate drainage of secretions; monitor output (bowel and bladder); provide contact with parents.

Multiple choice

1. d;   2. a;   3. c;   4. d;   5. b;   6. a;   7. d;
8. c;   9. b;   10. c

Matching

1. A;   2. A;   3. B;   4. A;   5. B;   6. B;   7. A;
8. B

True and False

1. False.

   Decreased PaO$_2$ and decreased pH initiate respirations.

2. False.

   Inadequate glucuronyl transferase levels cause bilirubin to collect in neonate's tissues.

3. False.

   Blood glucose of 60 mg/ml.

4. True.

5. True.

6. False.

At birth, the newborn has low levels of all immunoglobulins. Elevated levels of IgM indicate a potential infection.

ANSWERS TO CHAPTER 31

Key terms

1. D; 2. H; 3. E; 4. I; 5. F; 6. O; 7. A;
8. K; 9. M; 10. B; 11. J; 12. C; 13. G. 14. N;
15. L

Short answers

1. 65 to 70%.

2. Fomites.

3. 30.

4. Hypoglycemia.

5. Head or face.

6. Bilirubin.

7. Cold.

8. Sterile water is used to asses the patency of the gastrointestinal system. If the infant were to aspirate the first feeding, sterile water would be the least noxious substance introduced.

9. When a Yellen clamp is used a surgical probe separates the glans from the prepuce and then the clamp is applied over the prepuce which has been stretched. Pressure is sufficient to cut all the blood vessels and after 3-5 minutes the clamp is cut off with a scalpel. Generally, anesthesia is not used. Use of the Plastibell is somewhat less traumatic. The prepuce and the glans are separated and the Plastibell is positioned over the glans. A suture is tied at the base of the Plastibell to ligate the blood vessels and the distal portion of the prepuce is cut off with a scalpel. The Plastibell will fall off in 2-3 days when healing has occurred. Anesthesia is not usually used. Both procedures are surgical procedures.

ANSWERS TO CHAPTER 31

10.
- a. The room should be 75-80°F and free from drafts.
- b. No. It is not necessary to retract the foreskin for the first 3-6 months of life and the foreskin is only retractable in 50% of males at 1 year of life.
- c. No. The baby may not have a tub bath until the cord has fallen off, which is usually about 7-10 days of life.
- d. Automobile accidents are the leading cause of infant death. Most states now have mandatory car seat laws and it is necessary for you to have a car seat to take the baby home.
- e. You may have problems waking the baby; the baby may have a temperature 100°F; may be vomiting, have diarrhea, or a loss of appetite. Call your health care provider if the baby exhibits these symptoms.

Multiple choice

1. d;   2. b;   3. c;   4. b;   5. d

Matching

1. C;   2. D;   3. B;   4. A;   5. F;   6. E

True and False

1. False.

   The birthing room or labor-delivery-recovery-postpartum (LDRP) room contains the whole process in one room.

2. True.

3. False.

   The diagnostic problem category of ineffective thermoregulation is often an priority area for intervention in the transitional period.

4. True.

5. False.

   Signs and symptoms of illness should always be included in a parent teaching discharge plan. Other children in the home is not a reliable indicator that parent's knowledge base is complete.

6. True.

7. True.

8. False.

   The number of visitors in the nursery must be limited. Handwashing is essential.

ANSWERS TO CHAPTER 32

Key Terms

1. E;   2. K;   3. M;   4. O;   5. Q   6. F;   7. A;
8. L;   9. J;   10. G;   11. B;   12. H;   13. C;   14. I;
15. P;   16. N;   17. D

Short answers

1. Nasal flaring, increased respiratory rate, cyanosis, chest retractions, and an expiratory grunt.

2. Refusal of two or more feedings; absent or uncoordinated suck, swallow, or gag reflexes; projectile vomiting.

3. Hypoglycemia is manifest by jitteriness, lethargy, and associated low blood glucose levels. Hypocalcemia is manifested by jitteriness, twitching, heightened sensitivity to sensory stimuli. Symptoms may progress into muscle spasms and convulsions. Central nervous system irritability is manifested by jitteriness or seizure activity. Jitteriness can be dampened or stopped by holding/swaddling the infant.

4.
    a. The neonate has a strong, regular heart rate of over 100 bpm; has adequate respiratory effort; and responds quickly to stimulation. Major interventions are unnecessary. Close observations are continued.

    b. The neonate is mildly depressed and requires immediate assistance to establish and maintain effective respirations. The neonate appears cyanotic, with a decreased muscle tone and diminished respiratory effort. Heart rate is usually above 100 bpm. Gentle stimulation can be accomplished by briskly drying the neonate.

    c. The neonate is moderately depressed. The neonate appears cyanotic and flaccid and has weak, ineffective respirations. The heart rate is under 100 bpm. Immediate support is necessary to reverse the newborn's deteriorating condition.

    d. The neonate is severely depressed and requires maximum resuscitation efforts and support. The neonate is cyanotic and flaccid. There may be no respiratory effort or heart rate. Stimulation will not effect an improvement in the neonate's condition.

5. Lethargy, high-pitched cry, pupillary abnormalities and unusual eye movement, jitteriness seizure activity, and abnormal fontanelle size or bulging fontanelles.

Multiple choice

1. c;   2. a;   3. b;   4. c;   5. b

ANSWERS TO CHAPTER 33

Matching

1. E;   2. D;   3. C;   4. B;   5. A;   6. F

True and False

1. True.
2. False.

   Care cannot proceed until the nurse has identified all significant factors.

3. True.
4. True.
5. False.

   The nurse must include an ongoing evaluation of the parents responses to the high-risk infant.

ANSWERS TO CHAPTER 33

Key terms

1. J;   2. I;   3. H;   4. G;   5. F;   6. K;   7. E;
8. D;   9. C;   10. B;   11. A

Short answers

1.
   a. Prevention and early identification of physical complications.
   b. Assessment of extrauterine adaptation.
   c. Establishment of a feeding pattern.
   d. Support of parent-infant attachment.

2. Possible answers might include:
   a. Infiltration - observe for edema on neck or chest area; tape and restrain insertion site to prevent movement of catheter.
   b. Phlebitis - tubing and IV solution replaced every 24 hours using strict sterile technique; check site for evidence of erythema.
   c. Systemic infection - same as above.
   d. Accidental fluid overload - use minidrip tubing attached to fluid reservoir and an infusion pump.
   e. Air embolus - care must be taken when disconnecting lines to prevent introduction of air into system.

3. Infection, Thrombosis, Vasospasm, and Hemorrhage.

4. Possible answers might include:

   a. Examine IV site at least every hour for evidence of infiltration or inflammation.
   b. Be alert for signs of fluid imbalance.
   c. Maintain meticulous I & O records.
   d. Test urine for glucose and protein at least every 8-12 hours.
   e. Measure urine specific gravity.
   f. Assess for hyperbilirubiuema.
   g. Continuous IV infusion of insulin may be initiated for plasma glucose levels 250 mg/dl.

5.
   a. Increase in metabolic rate.
   b. Increase in oxygen consumption.
   c. Decrease in surfactant production.
   d. Hypoglycemia.

6. Possible answers might include:

   a. Very low birth weight/prematurity.
   b. Exchange transfusions.
   c. Intraventricular hemorrhages.
   d. Apnea.
   e. Sepsis.
   f. Patent ductus arteriosus with indomethacin administration.
   g. Vitamin E deficiency.

7. Possible answers might include:

   a. Impaired maternal blood flow through placenta.
   b. Impaired blood flow through umbilical cord.
   c. Impaired fetal circulation.
   d. Impaired respiratory effort.

8.
   a. Growth retardation.
   b. Microcephaly.
   c. Hepatosplenomegaly.

9. Blood, spinal fluid, and urine cultures. Gram stain of gastric aspirate may be done immediately after birth. Cultures axilla, groin, rectum, and nasopharynx are performed when amnionitis is suspected after prolonged rupture of membranes.

ANSWERS TO CHAPTER 34

10. Seizure activity, hypotonia, bulging fontanelles, unusual posturing, depressed cardiac/respiratory function, and hypothermia.

Multiple choice

1. c;   2. b;   3. c;   4. d;   5. c;   6. b;   7. b;
8. a;   9. c;   10. a

Matching

1. C;   2. A;   3. D;   4. B

True and False

1. True
2. False.
   Parents need lots of education to care for high-risk infants at home.
3. True.
4. True.
5. False.
   The infant is usually LGA.
6. True.
7. True.
8. False.
   Mother is Rh negative and fetus is Rh positive.

ANSWERS TO CHAPTER 34

Key terms

1. C;   2. D;   3. A;   4. B

Short answers

1.
   a. Atrial Septal Defect.
   b. Ventral Septal Defect.
   c. Patent Ductus Arteriosus.
   d. Phenylketonuria.
   e. Maple Syrup Urine Disease.

2.
   a. Emphasize the infant's inability to metabolize phenylalanine, a protein found in many food sources. Alleviate maternal guilt feelings and her diet has not effect upon the condition.
   b. The prognosis for children with PKU is very good when diet is started before 1 month of age and the diet is followed very closely to keep the phenylanine at a safe level. This is a treatable disease with the goal of promoting normal development.
   c. PKU is not an allergic reaction. The baby cannot break down one specific protein found in milk and certain other food products.

3. This keeps pressure off the open defect and prevents further neurologic damage and tissue breakdown.

4. To decompress the stomach and lessen the degree of ventilatory compromise.

5. Helps prevent accumulation of pulmonary secretions and helps minimize risk of respiratory infection.

6. A picture promotes bonding.

7. To document alteration in bowel elimination. Vomitus may be bile-colored with an intestinal obstruction; if not patent, abdominal distension may occur since gas and stool cannot be eliminated.

Multiple choice

1. d;   2. c;   3. b;   4. a;   5. c;   6. c

Matching

1. B;   2. A;   3. B;   4. A;   5. B;   6. B;   7. A

ANSWERS TO CHAPTER 35

True and False

1. True.
2. False.
   They begin vomiting in the 3rd to 5th week of life.
3. False.
   To the right of the umbilical cord.
4. True.
5. True.
6. False.
   It is commonly associated; approximately 80% of all cases.
7. True.
8. False.
   It is a left-to-right shunt.
9. False.
   46 chromosomes.
10. True.

ANSWERS TO CHAPTER 35

Key terms

1. F;   2. D;   3. H;   4. G;   5. C;   6. B;   7. E;
8. A

Short answers

1. Breastfed infants have lower rates of infections due to immunologic properties of breast milk. Breastfeeding may help in preventing development of allergies in the infant. Breast milk contains epidermal growth factor (EGF) which promotes cellular growth. Breastfeeding enhances the return of the mother's body to its non-pregnant state. A close emotional bond develops between the mother and her breastfed infant.

2. In general, infants gradually increase the amount taken at each feeding while slowing decreasing the number of feedings in a 24 hour period. From birth to 2 weeks, the infant should take 2-3 oz. every 2 1/2 to 4 hours. From 2-4 weeks, the infant usually increases intake to 3-4 oz. every 3-4 hours. From 1 to 3 months, infants require 5 to 6 oz. per feeding about every 4-5 hours. For 3 to 7 months, infants take 6-7 oz. per feeding and are usually fed every 5-6 hours. From 7 to 12 months, formula needs are met in 3 to 4 feedings, usually at meal times and bedtime, with 7-8 oz. taken at each feeding.

3. 9 bread group servings

   4 vegetable group servings

   3 fruit group servings

   3 milk group servings

   6 meat group servings (ounces)

   73 total fat (grams)

   12 total added sugars (teaspoons).

4. Possible answers might include:

   a. Steady increase in weight and length/height.

   b. Regular patterns of activity and sleep.

   c. In general, a happy disposition.

   d. Overall appearance of appropriate weight for length with firm muscles and presence of subcutaneous fat.

   e. Doubles weight by six months.

   f. Teeth erupt by 5-6 months.

Multiple choice

1. b;   2. c;   3. d

Matching

1. A;   2. B;   3. A;   4. B;   5. B;   6. A

True and False

1. False.

   It has declined again.

2. True.

3. True.

4. False.

   She does have special needs to meet higher than normal energy requirements.

ANSWERS TO CHAPTER 36

Key terms

1. G;   2. F;   3. B;   4. C;   5. E;   6. D;   7. A.

Short answers

1. Acquaintance.

2. Temperament.

3.
   a. Abdominal spasms and rigidity.
   b. Abdominal pain.
   c. Persistent unexplained and inconsolable crying.
   d. Move rapidly in and out of sleep.
   e. Irritable behaviors while feeding.
   f. Excessive activity.

4. Possible answers might include:
   a. Sleepy newborn.
   b. Poor feeder.
   c. Rigid body tone, non-cuddly.
   d. Infant who reacts strongly to stimuli, particularly mild or minimal stimuli.
   e. Infant who is not easily consolable.
   f. Irregular sleep-wake patterns.

5.
   a. Emotional abuse refers to the habitual verbal harassment of a child by disparagement, criticism, threat, and ridicule.
   b. Neglect comprises a lack of physical caretaking and supervision.
   c. Physical abuse can be defined as harm or threatened harm suffered by a child through nonaccidental injury or poisoning as a result of acts or deliberate omission by the caretaker.
   d. Sexual abuse is the involvement of dependent; developmentally immature children in sexual activity.

Multiple choice

1. c;   2. a;   3. c;   4. b

Matching

1. C;   2. C;   3. D;   4. A;   5. B;   6. F;   7. E;
8. B

True and False

1. True.
2. True.
3. False.

    There are many types of families from a variety of cultures and all care must be individualized.

4. True.